# Orthodontic and Surgical Managem<

# Orthodontic and Surgical Management of
# IMPACTED TEETH

## Vincent G. Kokich, DDS, MSD
Affiliate Professor
Department of Orthodontics
University of Washington School of Dentistry
Seattle, Washington

## David P. Mathews, DDS
Affiliate Associate Professor
Department of Periodontics
University of Washington School of Dentistry
Seattle, Washington

Private practice
Tacoma, Washington

**Quintessence Publishing Co, Inc**

Chicago, Berlin, Tokyo, London, Paris, Milan, Barcelona, Beijing,
Istanbul, Moscow, New Delhi, Prague, São Paulo, Seoul, Singapore,
and Warsaw

**Library of Congress Cataloging-in-Publication Data**

Kokich, Vincent G., author.
 Orthodontic and surgical management of impacted teeth / Vincent G. Kokich Sr, David P. Mathews.
       p. ; cm.
 Includes bibliographical references and index.
 ISBN 978-0-86715-445-0 (softcover)
 I. Mathews, David P., author. II. Title.
 [DNLM: 1. Tooth, Impacted--surgery. 2. Oral Surgical Procedures--methods. 3. Ortho-dontics--methods. WU 600]
 RK521
 617.6'43--dc23
                               2013039998

© 2014 Quintessence Publishing Co, Inc

Quintessence Publishing Co, Inc
4350 Chandler Drive
Hanover Park, IL 60133
www.quintpub.com

5 4 3 2 1

Editor: Leah Huffman
Design: Ted Pereda
Production: Angelina Sanchez

Printed in China

# Contents

Preface *vii*

**1** **Impacted Maxillary Central Incisors** *1*

**2** **Labially Impacted Maxillary Canines** *27*

**3** **Palatally Impacted Canines** *71*

**4** **Impacted Mandibular Canines** *103*

**5** **Impacted Premolars** *115*

**6** **Impacted Mandibular Molars** *141*

**7** **Complications and Adverse Sequelae** *155*

Index *173*

# Preface

This publication is the culmination of Vince's vision to write a book chronicling our 39 years of working together in an interdisciplinary manner, treating patients with impacted teeth. There has been very little written on this subject. Vince was the premier educator in orthodontics, and he felt very strongly that we should compile these cases in a very well-crafted book.

Sadly, he passed away before we were able to finish the last chapter. His longtime friend and colleague Dr Peter Shapiro; his son, Dr Vince Kokich, Jr; his daughter, Mary; and his wife, Marilyn, graciously helped me put the final touches on this fine work.

This book includes a chapter on every type of impaction an orthodontist and surgeon will encounter. It describes, in detail, the surgeries to uncover these impactions and the appropriate orthodontic mechanics to move these teeth once they are uncovered. It is the most complete, organized, and up-to-date book on this subject. It is ideal for orthodontists, pedodontists, periodontists, oral and maxillofacial surgeons, and general dentists who treat these types of cases.

We are fortunate to have so many fine orthodontists in Pierce County, Washington, who contributed to some of the cases in this book. They were all students of Vince's, and we are indebted to them for helping us leave this exceptional legacy.

Vince was the quintessential orthodontist/teacher in the world, and it is only fitting that Quintessence helped us bring this one of a kind book to fruition.

With heartfelt gratitude,
**David P. Mathews,** DDS

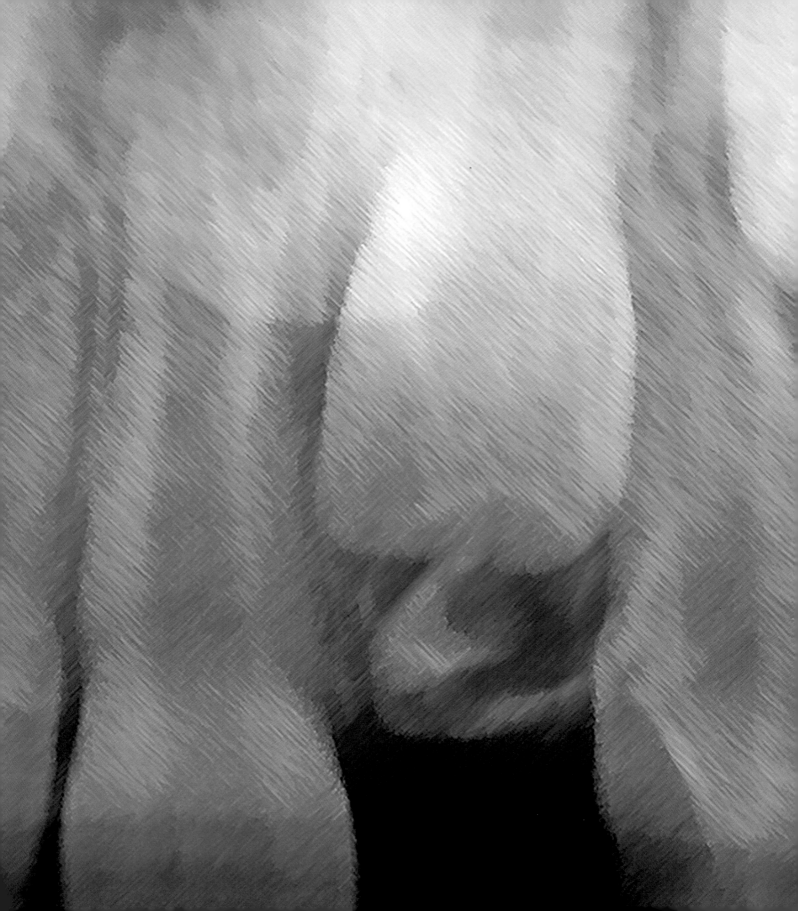

# Impacted Maxillary Central Incisors

## Etiology

The most commonly impacted teeth are the mandibular third molars, followed by the maxillary canines, mandibular second premolars, and maxillary central incisors.[1] Several causes of maxillary central incisor impaction have been documented, including crowding,[2] trauma,[3,4] root dilaceration,[5–9] presence of an odontoma,[10,11] presence of a dentigerous cyst,[12] or presence of a supernumerary tooth or mesiodens.[13–16] Some mesiodentes are located in the maxillary midline, between the two central incisors. In this situation, the supernumerary tooth is not blocking the path of eruption of the maxillary central incisors, and all anterior teeth potentially could erupt normally, including the mesiodens. The solution for this problem is to extract the mesiodens and close the space between the maxillary central incisors orthodontically. However, in most situations, when a mesiodens is present, it is positioned lateral to the maxillary midline and blocks the path of eruption of either the right or left central incisor. If multiple supernumerary teeth are present, both central incisors could become impacted (Fig 1-1).

## Fig 1-1 ) Multiple supernumerary teeth.

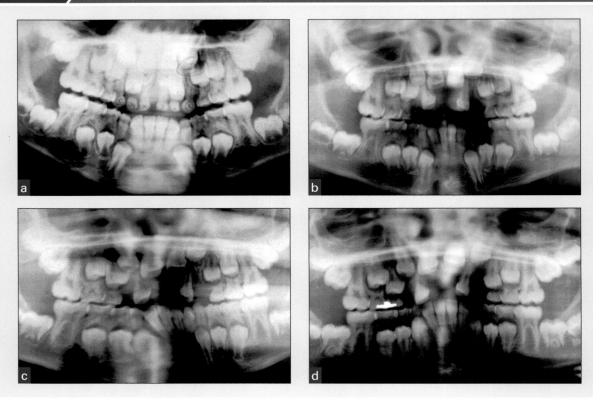

(a) This young patient had two supernumerary teeth that developed coronal to the maxillary central incisors. (b) The supernumerary teeth as well as all six maxillary anterior primary teeth were extracted to facilitate the eruption of the permanent maxillary incisors. (c and d) However, the follicles of the central incisors were damaged during the surgery, and, as a result, the lateral incisors erupted while the central incisors remained impacted.

If the supernumerary tooth or teeth are discovered early and extracted,[17] the central incisor could erupt spontaneously (see Fig 1-2). However, the method of extraction and extent of damage to the surrounding area could disrupt the natural eruption of the central incisor(s) and result in impaction. A series of articles published by Marks et al[18–22] emphasizes the importance of the integrity of the dental follicle during the normal eruptive process. In their experiments, the researchers intentionally and selectively damaged various parts of the developing tooth bud in an attempt to disrupt the eruptive process and cause impaction of the tooth. However, intentional injury to the root and various parts of the crown of the unerupted tooth did not prevent tooth eruption. But when the dental follicle was damaged or removed, eruption stopped. These researchers believe that the integrity of the dental follicle is critical to the normal eruption of any tooth.

Therefore, if the mesiodens or supernumerary tooth can be extracted without damaging the follicle of the subjacent central incisor, the impediment to eruption will be eradicated, and the impacted central incisor should erupt. This process is illustrated in Fig 1-2. This patient was 8 years old, and the maxillary left central incisor and both maxillary lateral incisors had erupted (see Fig 1-2a). However, the right central incisor had not erupted. A periapical radiograph revealed a supernumerary tooth that was apparently blocking the eruptive path of the right central incisor (see Fig 1-2b). A labial flap was elevated, and the supernumerary tooth was identified and removed without extracting the primary central incisor or damaging the follicle of the developing right central incisor. The flap was repositioned, and the teeth were allowed to erupt. After 1 year, the right central incisor had erupted spontaneously without orthodontic intervention (see Fig 1-2c). Therefore, if the supernumerary tooth is diagnosed early and removed surgically without compromising the follicle of the impacted central incisor, the submerged tooth should erupt spontaneously.

**Fig 1-2** Interceptive removal of a supernumerary tooth.

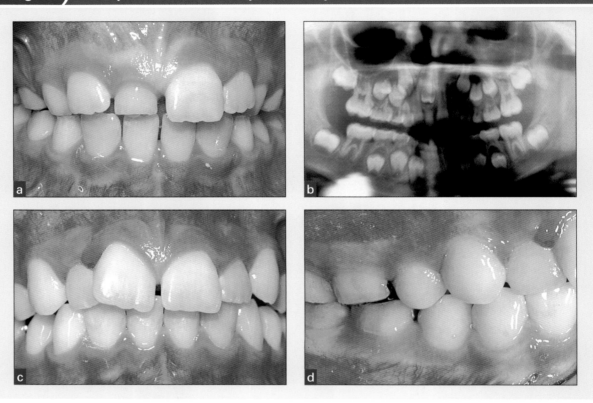

**(a)** This patient was 7 years, 8 months old. Her maxillary right central incisor was impacted within the alveolus. **(b)** The panoramic radiograph showed that a supernumerary tooth was blocking the path of eruption of the central incisor. The supernumerary tooth was removed without damaging the follicle of the right central incisor. **(c)** Eventually, the maxillary right central incisor erupted spontaneously without any further intervention. **(d)** This patient's occlusion was developing normally, and the parents chose not to proceed with any further orthodontic treatment.

However, in some situations, the proximity of the supernumerary tooth and the central incisor is so close that damage to the follicle of the impacted central incisor is unavoidable and inevitable. In other situations, an odontoma or dentigerous cyst may be present and in close proximity to the central incisor crown. Removal of the odontoma or cyst will usually damage the central incisor follicle, and the tooth will stop erupting. Finally, in some situations, a severely dilacerated root will cause impaction of the central incisor as a result of diversion of the tooth's eruptive path, placing it in an oblique position within the alveolus (see Fig 1-9). In all of these situations, it is best to uncover the impacted central incisor at the same time that the other surgery is being done, assuming the root of the central incisor is adequately developed.

# Preoperative Orthodontics

Usually, an impacted central incisor is recognized during the mixed dentition. At that time, all maxillary and mandibular central and lateral incisors are erupted, except for the impacted central incisor. The first step to facilitating spontaneous eruption is to extract any supernumerary teeth. If the tooth does not erupt autonomously, orthodontic treatment must be initiated to erupt the tooth.

Brackets should be placed on the remaining central incisor and the two maxillary lateral incisors. This bracket placement typically provides sufficient anchorage to erupt the impacted tooth. If the contralateral central incisor and adjacent lateral incisors are tipped toward one another, the space is opened using a compressed-coil spring. In this situation, it is necessary to place bands or brackets on the permanent maxillary first molars to provide anchorage during the course of orthodontic treatment.

After sufficient space has been established, a rectangular stabilizing wire is placed in the maxillary brackets. A loop may be placed in the archwire to temporarily anchor the attachment that will be placed on the impacted central incisor during the uncovering procedure. At this point, the patient is referred to the surgeon to uncover the impacted central incisor.

# Methods of Uncovering

There are four methods for uncovering an impacted maxillary central incisor: simple excision of tissue (gingivectomy), apically positioned flap (APF), the closed eruption technique, and surgical replantation. Central incisors are usually impacted labially. The apical location of the incisor will dictate the type of uncovering technique. Choosing the correct method will create the most stable and esthetic outcome after orthodontic eruption of the impacted tooth.

Most labially impacted central incisors are uncovered with the closed eruption technique.[23] Occasionally, the central incisor is located near or slightly coronal to the adjacent cementoenamel junction. If there is a wide zone of attached gingiva, a gingivectomy can be performed. The authors do not recommend an APF for uncovering maxillary central incisors because of the stability and esthetic problems associated with this technique.

## Gingivectomy

Gingivectomy can be performed if the resultant uncovering leaves at least 3 mm of gingiva around the exposed tooth. The gingivectomy should remove approximately two-thirds of the tissue covering the crown of the impacted tooth. A bracket and/or dressing can be placed to ensure that the tissue does not re-cover the tooth. There are few indications for this method of uncovering impacted maxillary central incisors. In most situations, the impacted tooth will be located at or above the mucogingival junction (Fig 1-3). If the tooth were at this level and an excisional approach were used, it would remove most of the gingiva, leaving inadequate attached gingiva over the labial portion of the crown (see Fig 1-3).

**Fig 1-3** Excisional uncovering (gingivectomy) of a maxillary left central incisor.

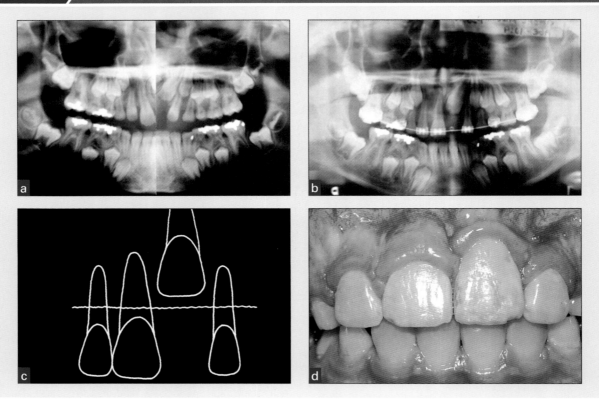

*(a)* The maxillary left central incisor in this 8½-year-old boy had not erupted. His occlusion was developing normally, but the right central incisor had drifted mesially. *(b)* Orthodontic alignment was initiated to create space for the impacted central incisor, but after 6 months, the tooth had not erupted. *(c)* A diagram shows that the incisal edge of the impacted central incisor was above the mucogingival junction. A gingivectomy was used to uncover the tooth, and it was erupted orthodontically into position. *(d)* After this phase of orthodontics, the gingival margin of the left central incisor was located apical to that of the right central incisor. In addition, the gingival margin of the left central incisor was thickened, rolled, and unesthetic.

## Apically positioned flap

A second type of surgical procedure for uncovering impacted maxillary central incisors is an APF (Figs 1-4 and 1-5). This procedure will create a predictable zone of attached gingiva, because it apically positions labial gingiva over the impacted central incisor. However, there are two problems associated with this technique: reintrusion and esthetics.[24] Therefore, the authors no longer use this technique to uncover maxillary central incisors.

If an APF were used to uncover a complex high labial impaction, it would be likely that gingival margin discrepancies would occur. This consequence is illustrated in Fig 1-4. The maxillary right central incisor has been moved into its proper location, but the gingival margin is more apical than that of the adjacent central incisor (see Figs 1-4f and 1-4g). This case illustrates one of the reasons why the closed eruption technique is used to uncover most labially impacted teeth: It maintains the original gingival architecture. An exception is the ectopic labially impacted tooth, which must remain uncovered after surgery. This situation requires an APF so that appropriate orthodontic mechanics can be applied to properly position the tooth.

## Fig 1-4 ) APF involving a horizontally impacted maxillary central incisor.

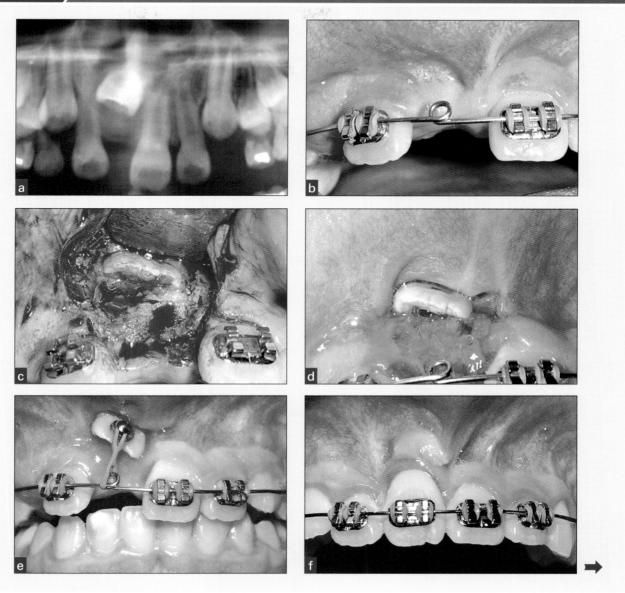

(a) The pretreatment radiograph shows the position of the impacted right central incisor, rotated 90 degrees. (b) Brackets were placed on the adjacent teeth, and sufficient space was created for the right central incisor. (c) An APF was reflected, bone was removed to uncover the crown, and the flap was sutured apically to leave the tooth uncovered. (d to f) Three weeks after uncovering, an elastomeric chain was used to erupt the right central incisor, and brackets were placed to position the crown and root of the formerly impacted central incisor.

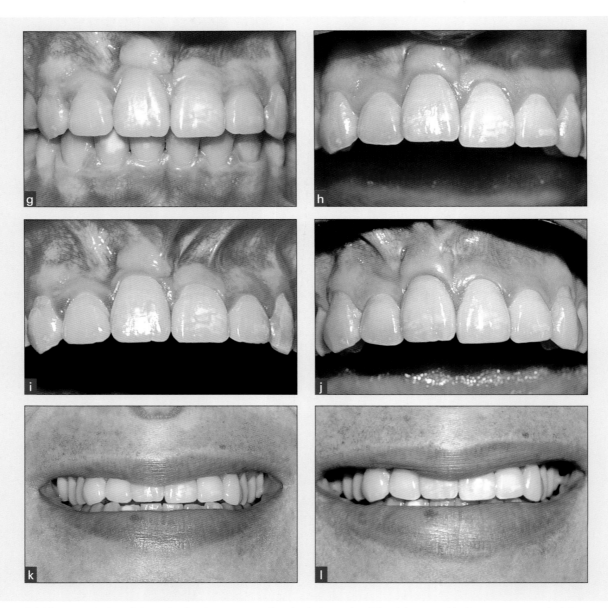

(g) After completion of the orthodontic treatment, the gingival margin of the right central incisor was more apical than that of the left central incisor. In addition, the gingiva was considerably thicker and unesthetic. (h) Five years after orthodontic treatment, the maxillary right central incisor had reintruded. This relapse was probably due to the pull of the mucosa (pseudofrena). (i) The tooth was re-treated to level the incisal edges. (j) Twenty-five years later, the right central incisor has reintruded, and the gingival margins are uneven again. (k and l) Five and 25 years after orthodontics, respectively, the incisal edge discrepancies are apparent when the patient smiles.

**Fig 1-5** APF to uncover two labially impacted central incisors.

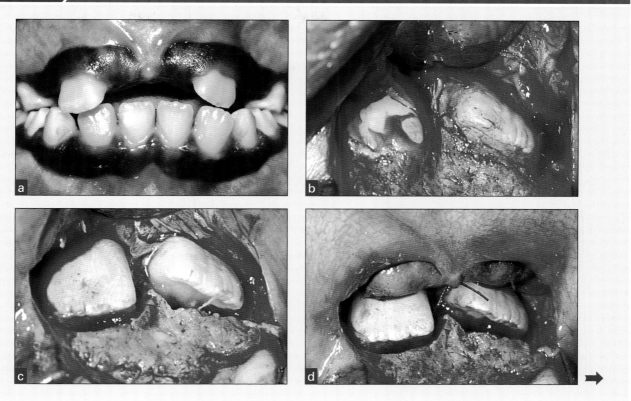

(a) One year after removal of supernumerary teeth, the permanent central incisors are still impacted. (b) A pedicle flap was reflected using midcrestal and vertical incisions, exposing the impacted central incisors. (c and d) Bone was removed to uncover the crowns of the two incisors, and the flap was apically positioned, leaving the incisors uncovered.

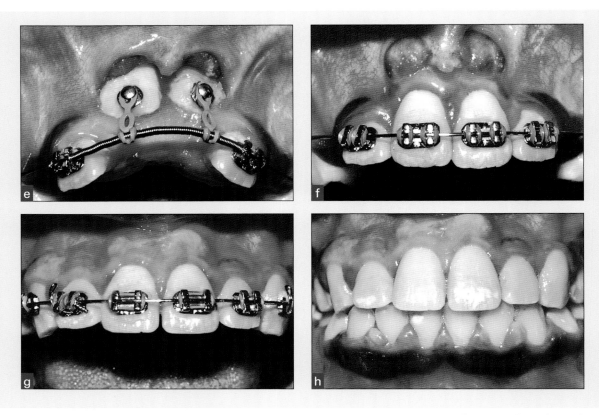

(e) Six weeks later, elastomeric chains were attached, and the eruption process was initiated. (f) One year later, the teeth were in ideal position. Note the bulky, apically displaced gingival tissue and disruption of the mucogingival junction. (g) Gingivoplasty was performed to eliminate the bulky tissue. Note the alteration of the natural pigmentation. (h) Two years later, the teeth have remained stable.

## Closed eruption technique

The third technique for uncovering an impacted maxillary central incisor is the closed eruption technique.[23–27] This technique involves reflecting a flap, uncovering the impacted tooth, placing an attachment, repositioning the flap, and erupting the tooth through the crest of the alveolar ridge (Figs 1-6 and 1-7). This technique results in the most natural-appearing gingiva over the erupted tooth.[25,28,29] The crown length is usually commensurate with the nonimpacted contralateral maxillary central incisor, resulting in a more esthetic result. The closed eruption technique also eliminates the reintrusion problem after the tooth has been erupted.

The closed eruption technique is illustrated in Fig 1-6. This patient had a supernumerary tooth coronal to the maxillary left central incisor (see Fig 1-6a). Brackets were placed on the erupted maxillary incisors, and space was apportioned for the impacted central incisor (see Figs 1-6b and 1-6c). A midcrestal incision was made in the edentulous ridge and joined with vertical incisions (see Fig 1-6d), and a full-thickness pedicle flap was reflected from the edentulous ridge. The supernumerary tooth was then located (see Fig 1-6e), but it communicated with the follicle of the impacted central incisor. The follicle was perforated when the supernumerary tooth was extracted (see Fig 1-6f). Because the follicle was disrupted, the central incisor would not erupt spontaneously, and therefore the impacted tooth was uncovered. There is usually a thin shell of bone covering part of the tooth. Approximately two-thirds of the crown was exposed with appropriate bone removal using curettes and surgical round burs. The area was isolated with hemostatic agents such as Surgicel (Ethicon) or Hemodent (Premier USA) cotton pledgets. The tooth was etched, and a bonding agent was placed. It is imperative that the field be kept clean and dry. With experience, hemostasis and a dry field can be accomplished in even the most difficult areas to access.

Once the bonding agent is placed and cured, the bonding process can continue. If the area gets contaminated with blood or debris after placement of the bonding agent, it can be cleaned with an alcohol wipe. At this point, a small cleat can be bonded to the tooth, and a chain can be ligated to the cleat. The chain can also be bonded directly to the tooth (see Fig 1-6g). The chain should have small enough links so the orthodontist can clip and remove one or two links as the tooth erupts. The chain should be malleable enough to avoid breakage but hard enough to avoid stretching as force is applied. Prefabricated chains with brackets for specific teeth are available (GAC International) and are easy to bond to impacted teeth. Fourteen-carat gold replacement chain with appropriate link size can also be effective. This can be purchased from a jeweler or pawnshop and is relatively inexpensive.

The pedicle flap is then returned to its original position and sutured. The chain is covered by the flap and exits at the midcrestal incision (see Fig 1-6h). The gold chain is ligated to the bracket on the adjacent tooth. A small ligating wire or an elastomeric ligature works well to fasten the chain to the bracket. The orthodontist may begin eruption of the tooth within 1 to 2 weeks.

**Fig 1-6** ) **Closed eruption technique.**

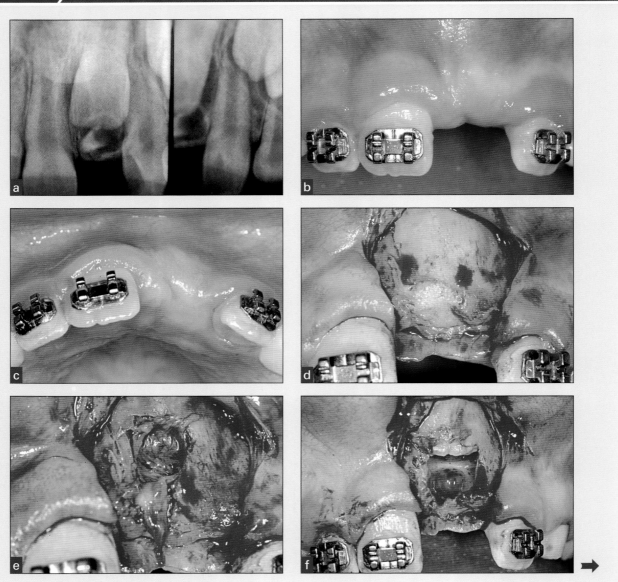

*(a)* The radiograph shows a supernumerary tooth and a labially impacted central incisor. *(b and c)* Brackets were placed, and appropriate space was created to allow eruption of the left central incisor. *(d)* A pedicle flap was reflected from the crest of the ridge. The supernumerary tooth and left central incisor were impacted within the alveolus and not visible. *(e)* A curette was used to remove the thin labial bone to find the supernumerary tooth. *(f)* The supernumerary tooth was removed, and the central incisor was now visible.

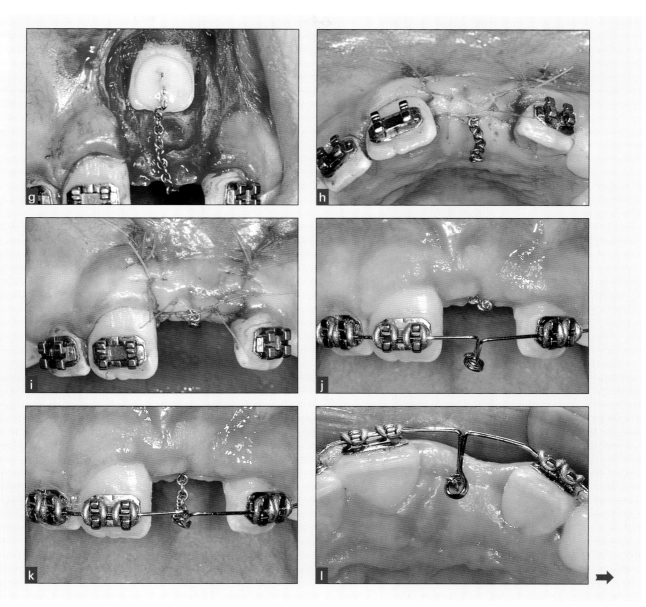

(g) Bone was removed from the crown of the central incisor, and a gold chain was bonded directly to the labial surface of the tooth. (h and i) The flap was repositioned and sutured. The chain exited through the incision at the midcrestal area. (j) Six weeks later, a Ballista spring was placed and was in the inactive state (ie, unattached). (k) The Ballista spring was activated and ligated to the gold chain. (l) The occlusal view of the activated spring demonstrates the midcrestal force.

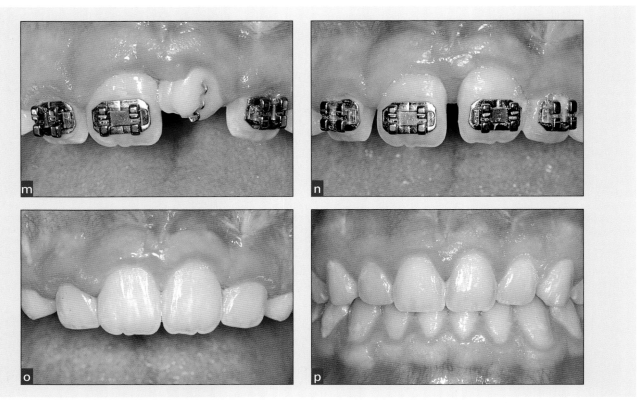

(m) The central incisor erupted through the crest of the ridge. The gingival margin was even with that of the right central incisor. (n) A bracket was placed for orthodontic finishing. (o) At completion, the tooth had a normal mucogingival junction and no pseudofrena. (p) Five years later, the gingival margins of the two central incisors are even and reintrusion has not occurred. (Orthodontics courtesy of Dr Vince Kokich, Jr, Tacoma, Washington.)

### Fig 1-7 ) Closed eruption technique involving a labially impacted maxillary central incisor.

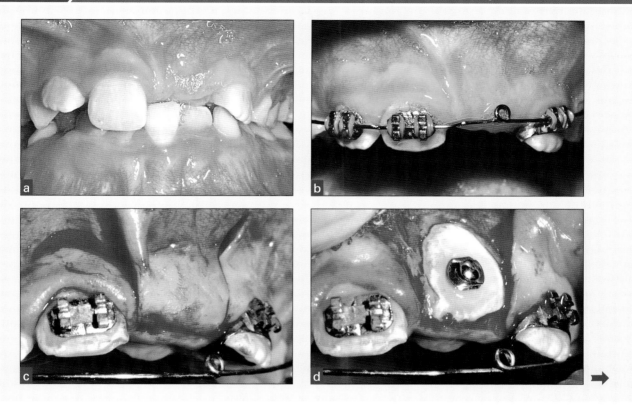

*(a)* This 10-year-old patient's left central incisor had not erupted. *(b)* Orthodontic treatment was initiated to create sufficient space between the right central and left lateral incisors. *(c and d)* A pedicle flap was reflected from the crest of the ridge, and a button was bonded to the labial of the impacted central incisor.

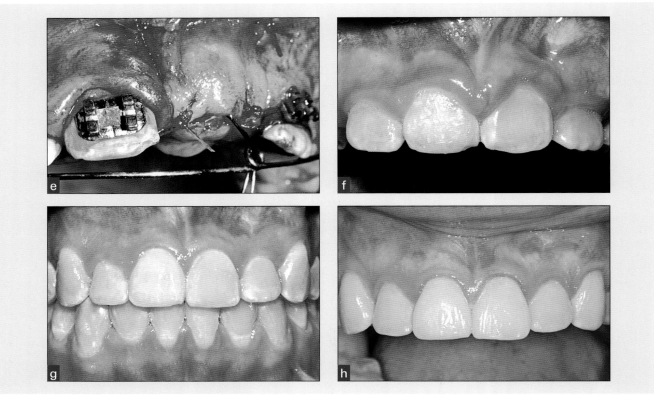

*(e)* The flap was repositioned and sutured, and elastomeric chains were used to erupt the tooth. *(f)* The central incisor was erupted orthodontically through the crest of the ridge. The gingival margins were at a commensurate level. *(g)* At the completion of the second phase of orthodontic treatment, the gingival margins of the two central incisors were at the same level. *(h)* Twenty-five years after orthodontic treatment, the gingival margins and incisal edges have remained stable.

The closed eruption technique can also be used when the tooth is impacted high in the vestibule on the labial aspect (Fig 1-8). In Fig 1-9, the maxillary right central incisor was impacted high in the vestibule near the base of the nasal spine. It was also positioned horizontally, which further complicated the surgical access (see Figs 1-9a and 1-9b). Initially, the maxillary incisors were banded (see Fig 1-9c) and the teeth were aligned, leaving a space for the impacted right central incisor (see Figs 1-9d and 1-9e). The patient was then ready to have the tooth uncovered. The use of an APF in this situation would be injudicious, so the authors chose the closed eruption technique.

**Fig 1-8** ) **Radiographic interpretation of an impacted central incisor.**

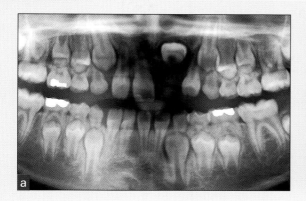 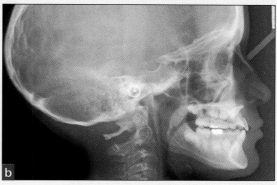

When a maxillary central incisor is impacted horizontally in the alveolus *(a)*, it is difficult to diagnose the orientation of the tooth root and crown with a panoramic radiograph. A cone beam image or a cephalometric radiograph *(b)* of the patient is helpful in identifying the position of the tooth prior to surgical uncovering.

A midcrestal incision was made, and a pedicle flap was reflected. Appropriate bone removal was accomplished, and the lingual surface of the tooth was visible. However, the labial aspect could not be accessed (see Fig 1-9f). A chain was then bonded to the lingual of the tooth, and the flap was returned to its original position. When the orthodontist applies appropriate force, the tooth will follow its normal eruptive pattern through the crest of the edentulous ridge, leaving adequate attached gingiva and a gingival margin that is esthetically harmonious with the adjacent central incisor. This type of complex impaction could also be treated by surgical replantation of the impacted central incisor.

### Fig 1-9 ) Closed eruption technique involving a horizontally impacted maxillary right central incisor.

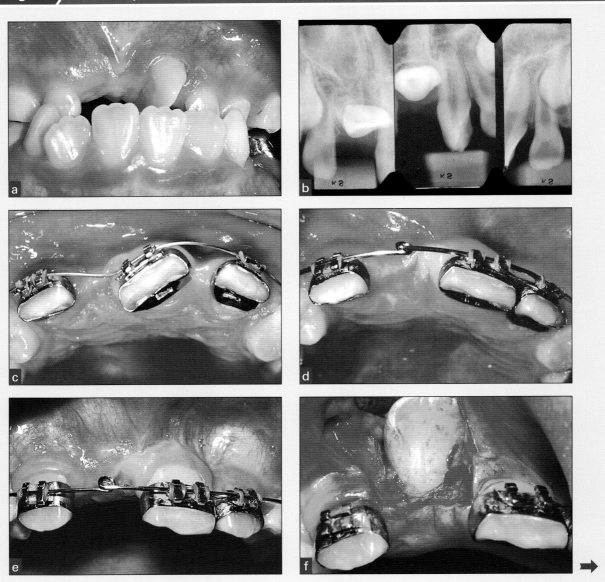

(a) The maxillary right central incisor was horizontally impacted and rotated 90 degrees, and the left central incisor was rotated and in lingual crossbite. (b) Pretreatment radiographs revealed that the right central incisor was horizontal and positioned toward the labial. (c to e) Brackets were placed, the teeth were aligned, and sufficient space was created for the impacted right central incisor. (f) A pedicle flap was reflected from the midcrest of the ridge, and the tooth was uncovered.

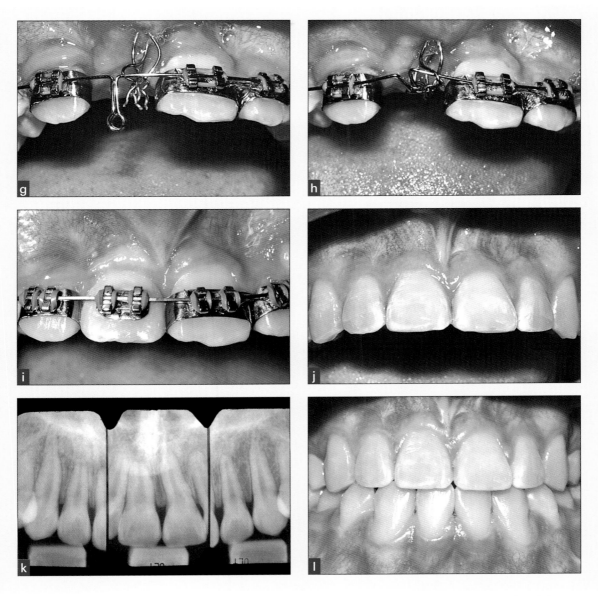

(g and h) A chain was attached and exited through the midcrestal incision area. A Ballista loop was used to deliver an eruptive force to the impacted central incisor. With the tooth in such a difficult position, it took 6 months to reorient the crown and root and erupt the tooth through the crest of the ridge. (i) After the tooth had erupted, a bracket was placed, and the tooth was aligned in its proper axial inclination. (j) After orthodontic treatment, the gingival margins were commensurate, and the gingiva and mucogingival junction were identical. (k) Five years later, a radiograph of the central incisors shows no root resorption. (l) After 5 years, the gingiva is esthetic, and reintrusion has not occurred.

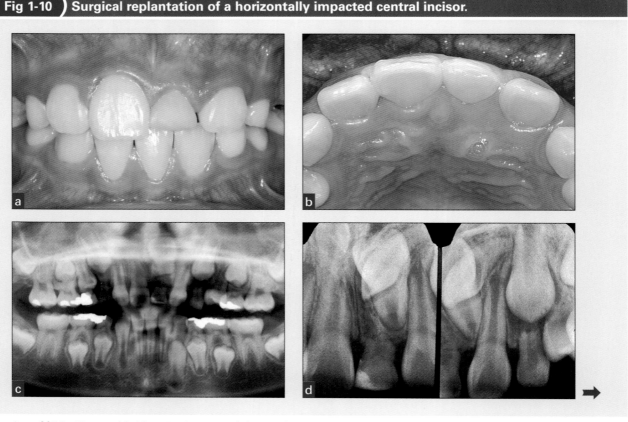

**Fig 1-10** ) **Surgical replantation of a horizontally impacted central incisor.**

*(a and b)* An 11-year-old girl retained a primary left central incisor. *(c and d)* The radiographs show that the right central incisor is horizontally impacted and rotated 90 degrees. In addition, there is a supernumerary tooth on the labial aspect of the impacted central incisor.

## Surgical replantation

The fourth technique for uncovering an impacted maxillary central incisor is surgical replantation.[30–35] This technique is reserved for those teeth that are severely rotated, either horizontally or vertically (Fig 1-10). Replanting these teeth in proper alignment will greatly facilitate the orthodontic movement. A full-thickness flap with appropriate vertical incisions is made (see Fig 1-10e). The impacted tooth is then uncovered carefully by removing the thin labial bone and exposing the entire follicle (see Fig 1-10f). The follicle of the impacted tooth is enucleated from its bony crypt (see Figs 1-10g and 1-10h). This is similar to removing the shell from a hard-boiled egg while keeping the egg completely intact, with no perforation in its delicate cover.

The edentulous area is prepared by creating a greenstick fracture of the labial plate and expanding it to create an osteotomy site for the follicle/tooth (see Fig 1-10i). The follicle/tooth unit is placed in the osteotomy site but in infraocclusion. The crown is bonded in place with a sturdy wire and dental composite (see Fig 1-10j). The flap is repositioned and sutured with 6-0 nylon. The repositioned tooth should be allowed to heal for 3 to 4 months before orthodontic treatment is initiated (see Fig 1-10l).

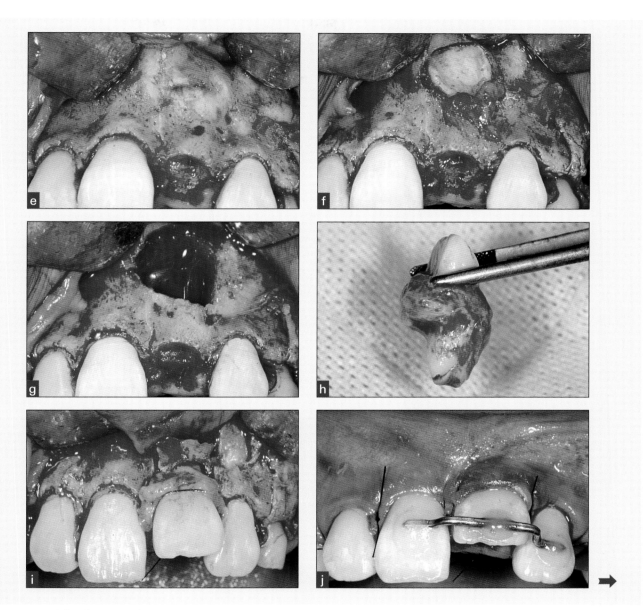

(*e and f*) A flap was reflected, and bone was removed carefully to expose the central incisor with its intact follicle. (*g to i*) The tooth, with its follicle, was enucleated and replanted in a proper vertical position. (*j*) The tooth was bonded in infraocclusion, and the flap was repositioned, leaving the tooth exposed. The supernumerary tooth was left intact as a backup in case the procedure failed.

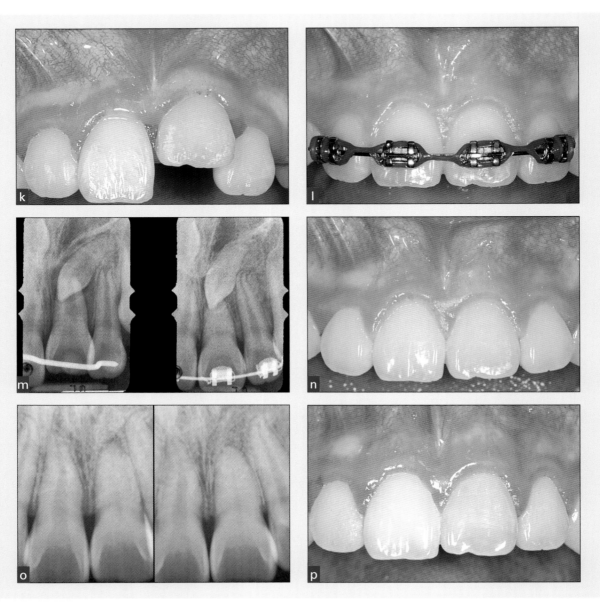

*(k)* Ten weeks later, orthodontic treatment was initiated. *(l)* One year later, orthodontic treatment was completed. *(m)* The radiograph taken after surgery *(left)* and the radiograph after 1 year *(right)* reveal the intact periodontal ligament of the central incisor without ankylosis. *(n)* One and a half years later, after completion of orthodontic treatment, the central incisors have esthetic gingival margins, and the incisal edges are at the same level. *(o and p)* Six years after the completion of orthodontics. (Courtesy of Dr Doug Knight [orthodontist] and Dr Jim Janakievski [periodontist], Tacoma, Washington.)

# Postoperative Orthodontics

During the postoperative orthodontic treatment phase, the key to success is erupting the maxillary central incisor into the center of the alveolar ridge. To accomplish this maneuver, the orthodontic force must originate from the center of the edentulous alveolar ridge. If the clinician directs the force labially toward the archwire, the impacted tooth may erupt into the oral cavity in a more labial position. This movement may cause apical positioning of the gingival margin over the erupted central incisor, creating a difference in the crown lengths between the impacted and nonimpacted central incisors, thus compromising the esthetic appearance of the teeth.[24]

To erupt the tooth into the center of the ridge, a Ballista loop is helpful[36] (see Figs 1-6j to 1-6l, 1-9g, and 1-9h). This loop can be activated, and its force is directed from the center of the ridge in a vertical direction (see Figs 1-6l and 1-9h). The size of the archwire typically used to create the Ballista loop is 0.018-inch stainless steel. This size of wire is large enough to avoid distortion and small enough to deliver a gentle force on the tooth. The end of the Ballista loop is ligated to the gold chain, which is bonded to the labial surface of the crown of the impacted tooth (see Fig 1-6k). As the tooth erupts (see Fig 1-6m), links of the chain are gradually removed, and the loop is once again secured to the impacted tooth. The length of the vertical portion of the loop is equal to the distance from the archwire to the center of the alveolar ridge. As the tooth is erupted, this type of loop will help pull the tooth into its normal path of eruption in the center of the ridge and not toward the labial. After the tooth has erupted, a bracket is bonded to the labial surface (see Fig 1-6n), and the crown and root of the tooth are positioned properly (see Figs 1-6o and 1-6p).

# Problems

Most problems in uncovering maxillary central incisors are related to improper soft tissue management and improper orthodontic mechanics. If a gingivectomy is performed in an inappropriate situation or the tooth is exposed through a small hole in the mucosa, there will be inadequate attached gingiva once the tooth is positioned orthodontically. This improper exposure could lead to gingival recession once the tooth is erupted. If this occurs on a central incisor, the gingival margins will be uneven, which could be an esthetic problem (see Fig 1-3d). Another problem with excisional uncovering of maxillary central incisors is stability. After simple excision of the mucosa overlying an impacted maxillary central incisor, the surrounding mucosa will form an epithelial attachment to the cementum of the root at that level. Therefore, as the tooth is erupted, an auxiliary or pseudofrenum will develop between the initial point of uncovering and the final position of the tooth within the alveolus. These pseudofrena may cause intrusion of the tooth because of their connection to the overlying mucosa. In some cases, the tooth could intrude 2 to 3 mm. This also occurs when the APF technique is used.

Improper access during surgery can lead to damage to the impacted tooth or adjacent teeth. Also, with improper access and visibility, appropriate bone removal is difficult. If the tooth is not uncovered adequately, the orthodontist will have difficulty moving it. Improper tooth isolation makes adequate placement of a bracket or chain more difficult. If there were a weak bond, the bracket or chain could debond during the orthodontic movement. This could necessitate a surgical procedure to reattach the appliance.

If an APF is used in an inappropriate situation, three undesirable sequelae could occur. First, if the tooth is impacted above the mucogingival junction (see Fig 1-4a), the clinical crown length of the impacted tooth would be longer than the adjacent central incisor (see Fig 1-4f). Although the cause of this problem is not known, it is probably related to a more rapid migration of the gingival margin apically during the eruption process. Increased crown length is a typical and consistent finding with the APF technique. Second, the erupted tooth could reintrude (see Figs 1-4g to 1-4l). As mentioned previously, this type of relapse is due to healing of the flap to the adjacent mucosa when it is positioned apically over the root of the impacted tooth. As the tooth erupts, the adjacent mucosa is drawn coronally, creating pseudofrena that tend to distract the tooth apically with time. Third, impactions located near the nasal spine are extremely difficult to leave uncovered when an APF is used (see Figs 1-4d and 1-5d).

# References

1. Hou R, Kong L, Ao J, et al. Investigation of impacted permanent teeth except the third molar in Chinese patients through an x-ray study. J Oral Maxillofac Surg 2010;68:762–767.

2. Tanaka E, Hasegawa T, Hanaoka K, et al. Severe crowding and a dilacerated maxillary central incisor in an adolescent. Angle Orthod 2006;76:510–518.

3. Macías E, de Carlos F, Cobo J. Posttraumatic impaction of both maxillary central incisors. Am J Orthod Dentofacial Orthop 2003;124:331–338.

4. de Oliveira Ruellas AC, de Oliveira AM, Pithon MM. Transposition of a canine to the extraction site of a dilacerated maxillary central incisor. Am J Orthod Dentofacial Orthop 2009;135(4 suppl): S133–S139.

5. Chew MT, Ong MM. Orthodontic-surgical management of an impacted dilacerated maxillary central incisor: A clinical case report. Pediatr Dent 2004;26:341–344.

6. Cozza P, Marino A, Condo R. Orthodontic treatment of an impacted dilacerated maxillary incisor: A case report. J Clin Pediatr Dent 2005;30:93–97.

7. Farronato G, Maspero C, Farronato D. Orthodontic movement of a dilacerated maxillary incisor in mixed dentition treatment. Dent Traumatol 2009;25:451–456.

8. Hegde C, Hegde M, Parajuli U. Orthodontic repositioning of a malposed and dilacerated central incisor. Kathmandu Univ Med J 2009;7:435–437.

9. Neto J, Costa S, Estrela C. Orthodontic-surgical-endodontic management of unerupted maxillary central incisor with distoangular root dilaceration. J Endod 2010;4:755–759.

10. Batra P, Duggal R, Kharbanda OP, Parkash H. Orthodontic treatment of impacted anterior teeth due to odontomas: A report of two cases. J Clin Pediatr Dent 2004;28:289–294.

11. da Costa CT, Torriani DD, Torriani MA, da Silva RB. Central incisor impacted by an odontoma. J Contemp Dent Pract 2008;9:122–128.

12. Sharma D, Garg S, Singh G, Shveta S. Trauma-induced dentigerous cyst involving an inverted impacted mesiodens: Case report. Dent Traumatol 2010;26:289–291.

13. Moraes RS, Farinhas JA, Gleiser R, Primo LG. Delayed eruption of maxillary permanent central incisors as a consequence of mesiodens: A surgical re-treatment approach. J Clin Pediatr Dent 2004;28:195–198.

14. Bayram M, Ozer M, Sener I. Bilaterally impacted maxillary central incisors: Surgical exposure and orthodontic treatment: A case report. J Contemp Dent Pract 2006;7:98–105.

15. Kolokitha OE, Papadopoulou AK. Impaction and apical root angulation of the maxillary central incisors due to supernumerary teeth: Combined surgical and orthodontic treatment. Am J Orthod Dentofacial Orthop 2008;134:153–160.

16. Fujita Y, Takahashi T, Maki K. Orthodontic treatment for an unerupted and severely rotated maxillary central incisor. A case report. Eur J Paediatr Dent 2008;9:43–47.

17. Baart JA, Groenewegen BT, Verloop MA. Correlations between the presence of a mesiodens and position abnormalities, diastemas, and eruption disturbances of maxillary frontal teeth. Ned Tijdschr Tandheelkd 2009;116:399–402.

18. Cahill D, Marks S Jr. Tooth eruption: Evidence for the central role of the dental follicle. J Oral Pathol 1980;9:189–200.

19. Marks S Jr, Cahill D, Wise G. The cytology of the dental follicle and adjacent alveolar bone during tooth eruption in the dog. Am J Anat 1983;168:277–289.

20. Marks S Jr, Cahill D. Experimental study in the dog of the non-active role of the tooth in the eruptive process. Arch Oral Biol 1984;29:311–322.

21. Marks S Jr, Cahill D. Regional control by the dental follicle of alterations in alveolar bone metabolism during tooth eruption. J Oral Pathol 1987;16:164–169.

22. Marks S Jr, Schroeder H. Tooth eruption: Theories and facts. Anat Rec 1996;245:374–393.

23. Fournier A, Turcotte J, Bernard C. Orthodontic considerations in the treatment of maxillary impacted canines. Am J Orthod 1982;81:236–239.

24. Kokich VG, Mathews DP. Surgical and orthodontic management of impacted teeth. Dent Clin North Am 1993;37:181–204.

25. Vermette ME, Kokich VG, Kennedy DB. Uncovering labially impacted teeth: Apically positioned flap and closed-eruption techniques. Angle Orthod 1995;65:23–32.

26. Keijirou K, Kai H. Esthetic management of an unerupted maxillary central incisor with a closed-eruption technique. Am J Orthod Dentofacial Orthop 2000;118:224–228.

27. Becker A, Brin I, Ben-Bassat Y, Zilberman Y, Chaushu S. Closed-eruption surgical technique for impacted maxillary incisors: A postorthodontic periodontal evaluation. Am J Orthod Dentofacial Orthop 2002;122:9–14.

28. Chaushu S, Brin I, Ben-Bassat Y, Zilberman Y, Becker A. Periodontal status following surgical-orthodontic alignment of impacted central incisors with an open-eruption technique. Eur J Orthod 2003;25:579–584.

29. Chaushu S, Dykstein M, Ben-Bassat Y, Becker A. Periodontal status of impacted maxillary incisors uncovered by 2 different surgical techniques. J Oral Maxillofac Surg 2009;67:120–124.

30. Chaushu S, Zilberman Y, Becker A. Maxillary incisor impaction and its relationship to canine displacement. Am J Orthod Dentofacial Orthop 2003;124:144–150.

31. Tsai TP. Surgical repositioning of an impacted dilacerated incisor in the mixed dentition. J Am Dent Assoc 2002;133:61–66.

32. Agrait EM, Levy D, Gil M, Singh GD. Repositioning an inverted maxillary central incisor using a combination of replantation and orthodontic movement: A clinical case report. Pediatr Dent 2003;25:157–160.

33. Maia RL, Vieira AO. Autotransplantation of a central incisor with root dilaceration. Technical note. Int J Oral Maxillofac Surg 2005;34:89–91.

34. Janakievski J. Avulsed maxillary central incisors: The case for autotransplantation. Counterpoint. Am J Orthod Dentofacial Orthop 2012;142:9,11,13,15,17.

35. Kuroe K, Tomonari H, Soejima K, Maeda A. Surgical repositioning of a developing maxillary permanent central incisor in a horizontal position: Spontaneous eruption and root formation. Eur J Orthod 2006;28:206–209.

36. Jacoby H. The "ballista spring" system for impacted teeth. Am J Orthod 1979;75:143–151.

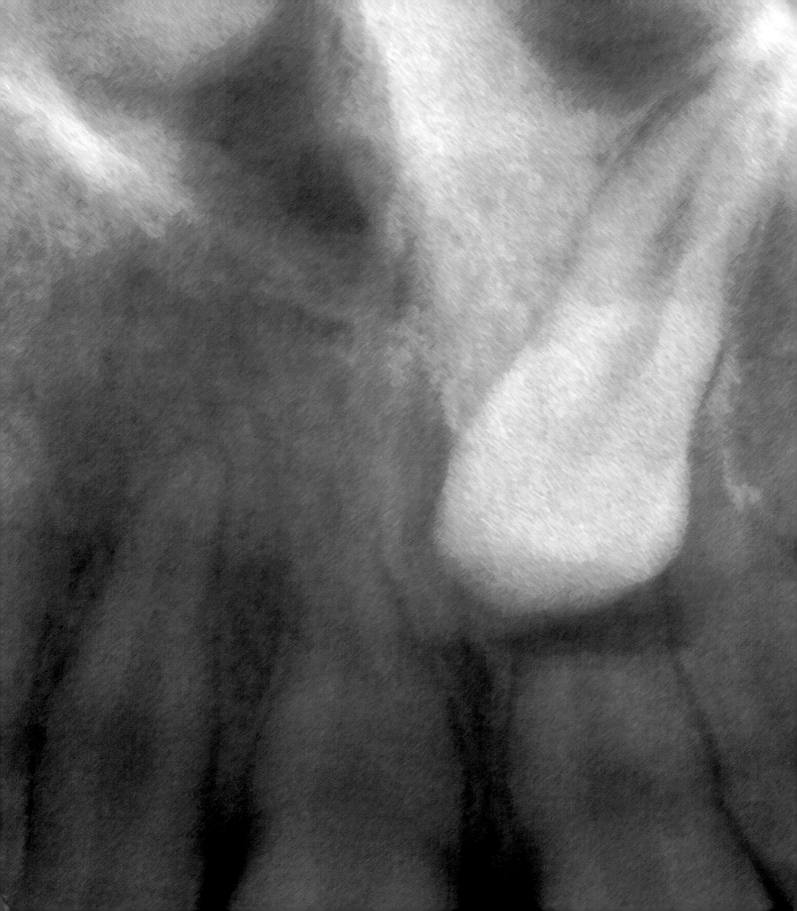

# Labially Impacted Maxillary Canines

## 2

After mandibular third molars, maxillary canines are the most commonly impacted teeth among patients referred for orthodontic treatment.[1] Previous studies have shown that while about two-thirds of maxillary canines are impacted palatally, one-third are impacted labially.[2] This chapter discusses the management of labial canine impactions. Labially impacted canines can be positioned ectopically, facial to the root of the lateral incisor, or they can be located in a midalveolar position. The location of the impaction will dictate the timing and type of surgery employed to uncover the tooth.

# Etiology

The etiology of labial impaction of a maxillary canine is likely to be multifactorial. It could be the result of ectopic migration of the canine crown over the root of the lateral incisor or shifting of the maxillary dental midline, which leads to insufficient space for the canine to erupt. Chung et al[3] have suggested that genetics plays a significant role in maxillary canine impaction. Others believe that genetic mechanisms strongly influence both the potential of the maxillary canine to be impacted and the guidance from the lateral incisor and that the stage of development plays a vital role in determining the ultimate position of the impacted canine.[4] On the other hand, Kim et al[5] found that the maxillary arch length, intermolar width, and palatal vault depth were associated with and played a role in the incidence of palatal versus labial impaction of maxillary canines. Similar findings were proposed by Yan et al,[6] who reported that the maxillary interpremolar width in the buccally impacted canine group was significantly smaller than that in the palatally impacted canine group.

# Interceptive Treatment

Interceptive treatment has been proposed by some researchers to promote self-correction and autonomous eruption of a labially impacted canine. Williams[7] has suggested that extraction of the maxillary primary canine as early as 8 or 9 years of age will enhance the eruption and self-correction of a labial or intra-alveolar maxillary canine impaction. Bonetti et al[8] found that extraction of both the primary canines and the primary first molars proved to be a more effective interceptive procedure compared with single canine extraction in improving the intraosseous position of an impacted canine.

Olive[9] has suggested that opening space for the canine crown with routine orthodontic mechanics may allow for spontaneous eruption of an impacted canine. O'Neill,[10] on the other hand, has shown that the prevalence rates for successful eruption of maxillary canines were significantly improved in patients who had palatal expansion to increase the maxillary arch length.

However, in some situations, even these techniques may not work, and the orthodontist will need to refer the patient to have the labial impaction uncovered surgically. There are three techniques for uncovering a labially impacted maxillary canine: excisional uncovering (Fig 2-1), an apically positioned flap (APF)[11] (Figs 2-2 and 2-3; see also Figs 2-6 to 2-11), and the closed eruption technique[12] (Fig 2-4; see also Fig 2-5).

**Fig 2-1** ) **Labially impacted maxillary right canine.**

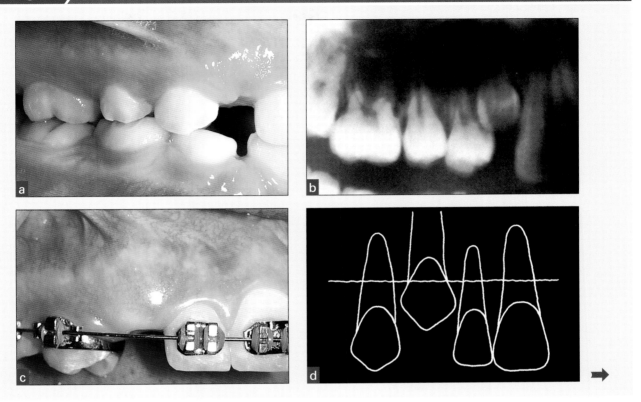

(a and b) All of the permanent teeth had erupted in this adolescent girl except for the maxillary right canine. (c) After initial orthodontic alignment, the tooth had still not erupted. (d) The canine crown was located toward the labial aspect, and most of the crown was coronal to the mucogingival junction.

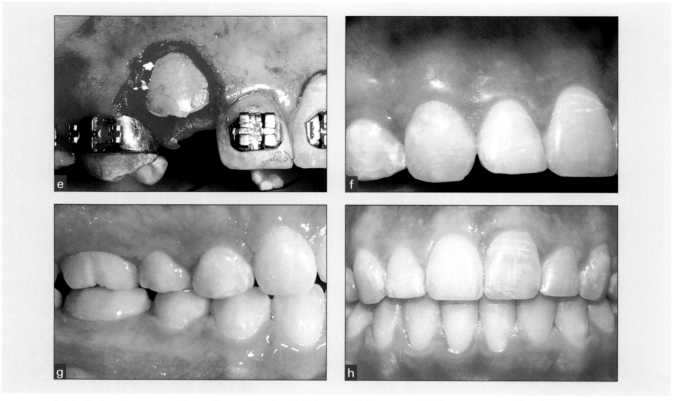

(e) A gingivectomy was performed, exposing the clinical crown of the canine. (f) After eruption and bracket removal, the gingiva and mucosa were stained with Schiller's solution to delineate the mucogingival junction. (g and h) The posttreatment photographs show that the gingival margin and width of gingiva of the previously impacted maxillary right canine are ideal and identical to the normally erupted left canine. (Figs 2-1c to 2-1f reprinted from Kokich[13] with permission.)

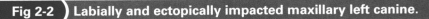

**Fig 2-2** ) **Labially and ectopically impacted maxillary left canine.**

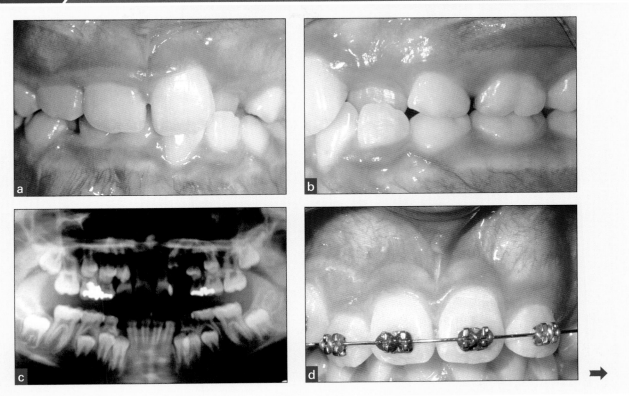

**(a and b)** This 10-year-old girl had a maxillary lateral incisor crossbite that had been treated with a first phase of orthodontics. When her remaining teeth had erupted, a second phase of treatment was started. **(c and d)** The maxillary left canine was impacted labially and ectopically positioned mesial to the root of the maxillary left lateral incisor.

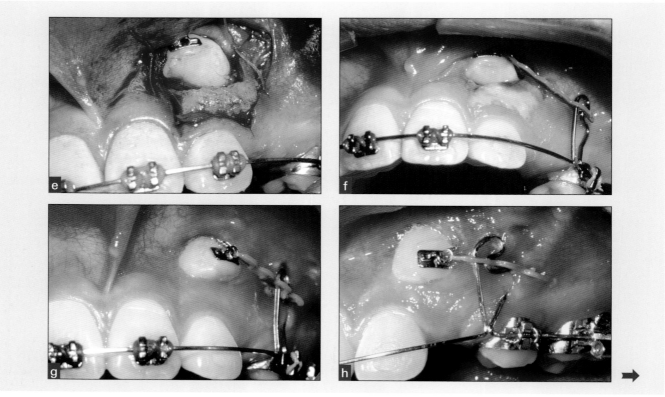

(*e*) A pedicle flap was reflected, leaving a collar of gingiva around the lateral incisor. After the crown was exposed, the flap was positioned apically, leaving the tooth uncovered. A gingival graft taken from the buccal of the first molar was placed over the lateral incisor to help prevent recession. (*f to i*) The bracket on the lateral incisor was removed to avoid contact between the canine crown and the lateral incisor root, and an auxiliary wire was extended apically into the vestibule to move the crown of the canine directly toward the distal to avoid damaging the bone labial to the lateral incisor.

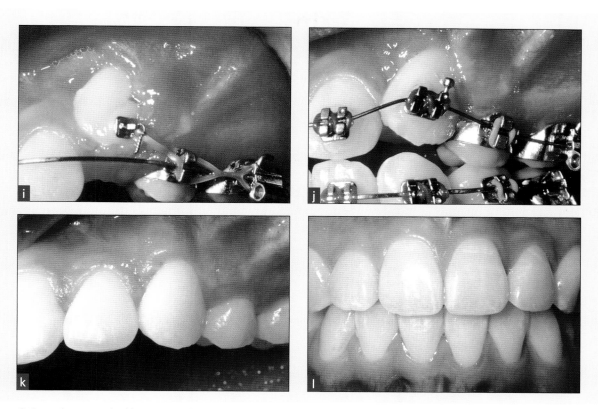

(j) Once the canine had been moved past the lateral incisor, the canine could be erupted vertically into the dental arch. (k and l) The posttreatment photographs show that the gingival levels of the canines and lateral incisors are identical to the contralateral side.

**Fig 2-3　Slightly labially impacted maxillary right canine.**

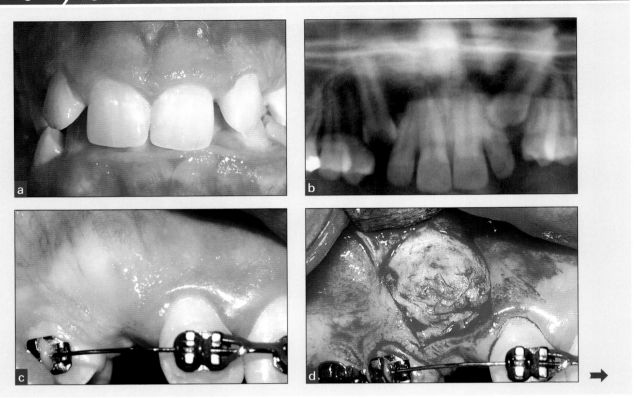

*(a)* This adolescent boy had a Class II, division 2 malocclusion requiring orthodontics, extraction of two mandibular premolars, and mandibular advancement surgery. *(b)* The maxillary right canine was impacted slightly labial to the middle of the alveolus and positioned near the mucogingival junction. *(c and d)* After initial orthodontic alignment of the maxillary arch, a pedicle flap was reflected and bone was removed to uncover the crown of the impacted canine.

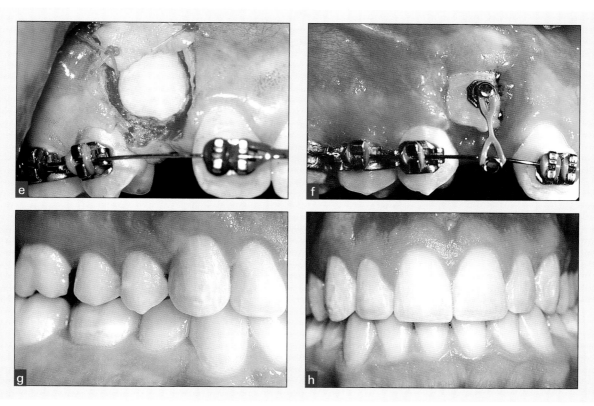

**(e)** The flap was apically positioned with resorbable sutures, exposing about two-thirds of the clinical crown. **(f)** Two months later, an eruptive force was placed on the tooth to move it into occlusion. **(g and h)** The posttreatment photographs show that the gingival levels of the maxillary canines are identical. This case also could have been treated with the closed eruption technique.

**Fig 2-4** **Impacted maxillary right canine erupted with a pin.**

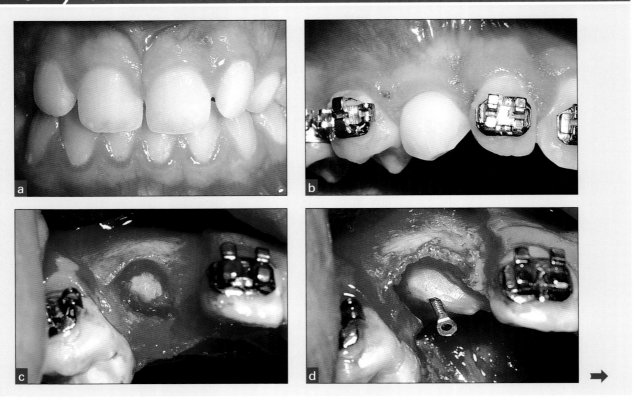

**(a)** The maxillary right canine in this 16-year-old girl was impacted in the midalveolar region, and the primary canine had not exfoliated. **(b)** After initial alignment of the maxillary teeth, the maxillary primary canine was extracted, but the permanent canine did not erupt. **(c and d)** Labial and palatal flaps were reflected, bone was removed to expose the incisal third of the permanent canine, and a pin was placed into the canine crown. The flaps were repositioned, leaving the pin exposed in the midcrestal area.

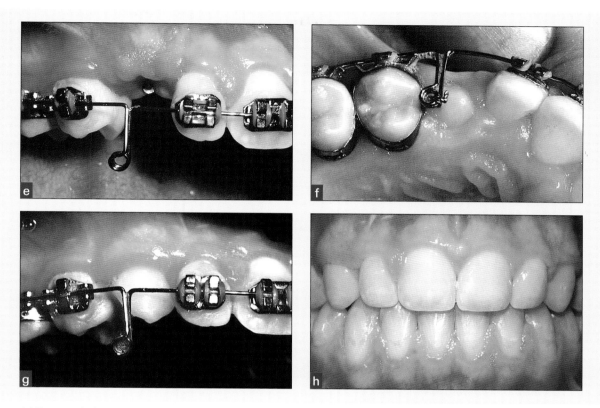

(e) Two months later, a Ballista spring was created in the maxillary archwire. (f) The spring was activated to deliver a vertical extrusive force to the canine. (g) With this technique, the crown typically erupts into the center of the alveolar ridge, similar to a naturally erupting tooth. (h) The posttreatment photograph shows that the gingival levels of the right and left canines are identical. This case was treated almost 40 years ago, and today a chain would be bonded to the incisal edge. (Reprinted from Kokich[13] with permission.)

# Choosing the Appropriate Uncovering Technique

Four criteria must be evaluated to determine the appropriate method for surgical uncovering[13]:

1. *The labiolingual position of the impacted canine crown.* If the tooth is impacted labially, then any of the three techniques could be used, because generally there is little, if any, bone covering the crown of the impacted canine. However, if the tooth is impacted within the center of the alveolus, then an excisional approach and an APF are not recommended, because extensive bone may need to be removed from the labial surface of the crown.

2. *The vertical position of the tooth relative to the mucogingival junction.* If the majority of the canine crown is positioned coronal to the mucogingival junction (see Fig 2-1), then any of the three techniques can be used. However, if the canine crown is positioned apical to the mucogingival junction (see Figs 2-2 and 2-3), then an excisional technique would be inappropriate, because it will result in a lack of gingiva over the labial of the tooth after it has erupted. In addition, if the crown is positioned significantly apical to the mucogingival junction (see Figs 2-6, 2-8, 2-11, and 2-12), then an APF also would not be appropriate, because it would result in instability of the crown and possible reintrusion of the tooth after orthodontics.[7] In the latter situation, a closed eruption technique will provide adequate gingiva over the crown and does not result in long-term reintrusion of the tooth.[8]

3. *The amount of gingiva in the area of the impacted canine.* If there is insufficient gingiva in the area of the canine (see Fig 2-3), then the only technique that will predictably produce more gingiva is an APF. However, if there is sufficient gingiva to provide at least 2 to 3 mm of attached gingiva over the canine crown after it erupts, then any of the three techniques could be used.

4. *The mesiodistal position of the canine crown.* If the crown is positioned mesially and over the root of the lateral incisor (see Figs 2-2, 2-6, and 2-10 to 2-12), then it could be difficult to move the tooth through the alveolus, unless it is completely exposed with an APF. In this latter situation, closed eruption or excisional uncovering generally would not be recommended.

An APF procedure should be used when the canine is impacted ectopically (ie, mesial to the lateral incisor or distal to the first premolar). This will allow the orthodontist access to apply appropriate mechanics to "jump" the tooth over the lateral incisor or premolar without damaging these adjacent teeth.

Some labially impacted teeth are located closer to the midalveolar position and are treated with the closed eruption technique. These are the easiest to access, so a chain can be bonded directly to the tooth to erupt the tooth through the crestal area. This movement mimics the natural eruption pathway the tooth would normally have taken (Fig 2-5).

**Fig 2-5** **Impacted maxillary right canine causing extensive root resorption.**

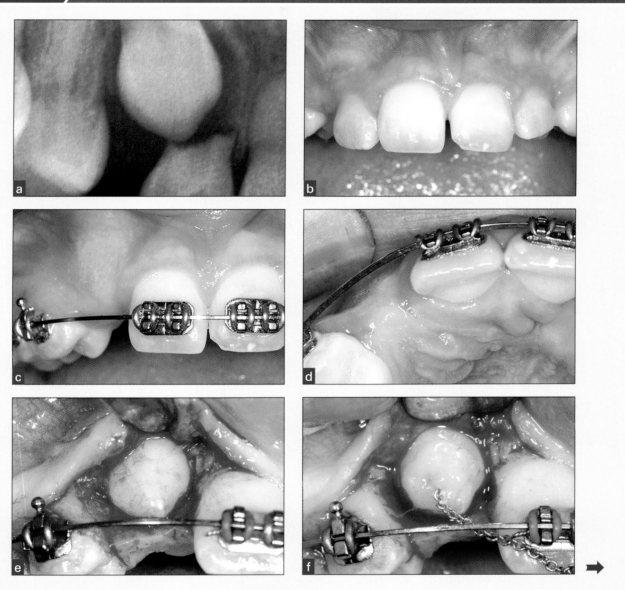

*(a and b)* The maxillary right canine in this adolescent girl had caused extensive resorption of the root of the right lateral incisor. The patient had arch length discrepancies in both dental arches and required tooth extraction. A similar resorptive problem had occurred on the contralateral maxillary lateral incisor, so the maxillary right and left lateral incisors and mandibular right and left first premolars were extracted. *(c and d)* Brackets were placed on all teeth, but after 6 months the maxillary right canine had not erupted. The closed eruption technique was employed to uncover the impacted canine. *(e and f)* A midcrestal incision was made, a labial flap was reflected to expose the crown, and a chain was bonded to the tooth.

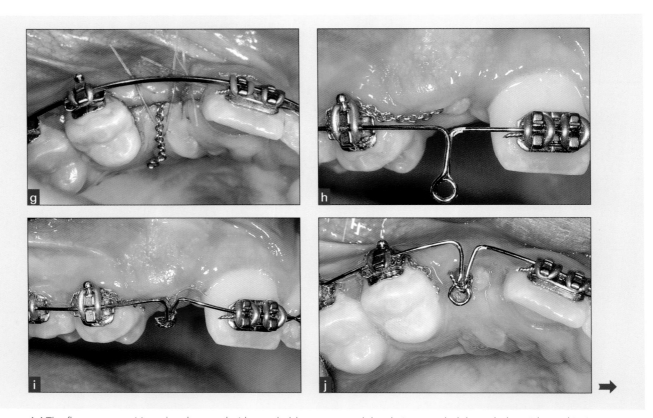

(g) The flap was repositioned and sutured with resorbable sutures, and the chain extended through the midcrestal incision. (h to k) A Ballista loop was created in 0.018-inch stainless steel archwire to deliver a vertical force in order to erupt the crown of the canine into the center of the alveolar ridge.

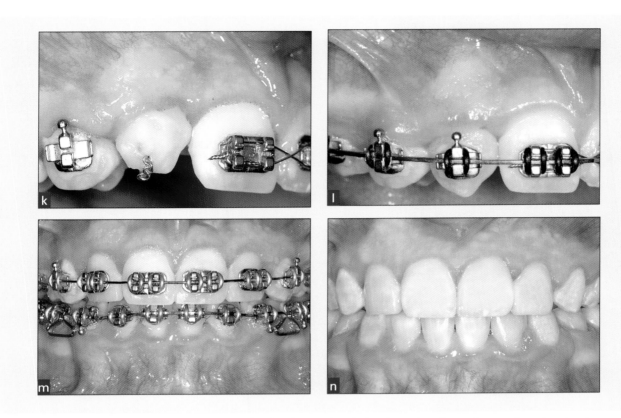

*(l to n)* After the tooth had erupted sufficiently, a bracket was bonded to the canine, the teeth were aligned, and restorative composite was bonded to the incisal edges of both canines to simulate the appearance of lateral incisors.

# Surgical Techniques

The labially impacted canine can be located ectopically or in its normal location. When it is ectopically impacted mesial to the lateral incisor or distal to the first premolar, it will be necessary to use the APF. This will allow the orthodontist access to apply appropriate mechanics to move the tooth past the lateral incisor or premolar without damaging the adjacent teeth (Fig 2-6).

**Fig 2-6** Impacted maxillary right canine erupted with a cleat and chain.

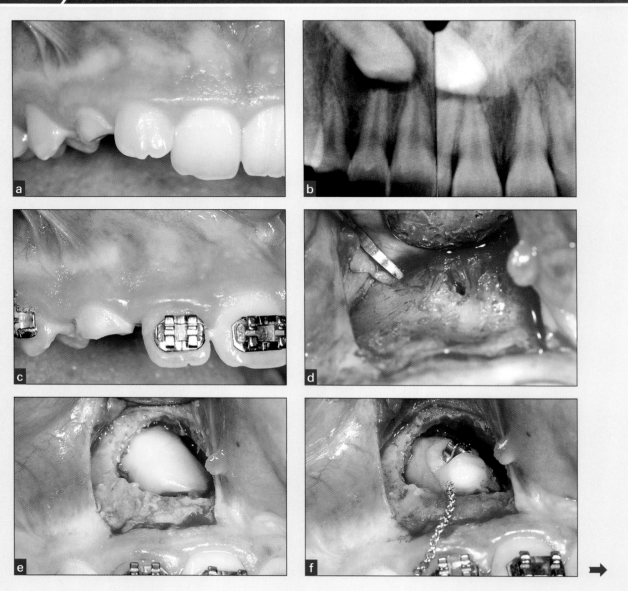

*(a)* The maxillary right canine was impacted in this adolescent girl. *(b)* The periapical radiographs show that the canine was positioned in the middle of the alveolus and slightly to the palatal. It had caused some resorption of the roots of the lateral and central incisors. However, palpation of the labial periapical region revealed that the crown of the canine could be accessed from a labial approach. *(c and d)* After initial orthodontic alignment, a pedicle flap was reflected from the labial of the central and lateral incisors, leaving a collar of gingiva on these teeth. *(e)* A window of bone was removed to expose about two-thirds of the crown of the impacted tooth. *(f)* A cleat with a separate auxiliary chain was bonded to the labial surface of the canine.

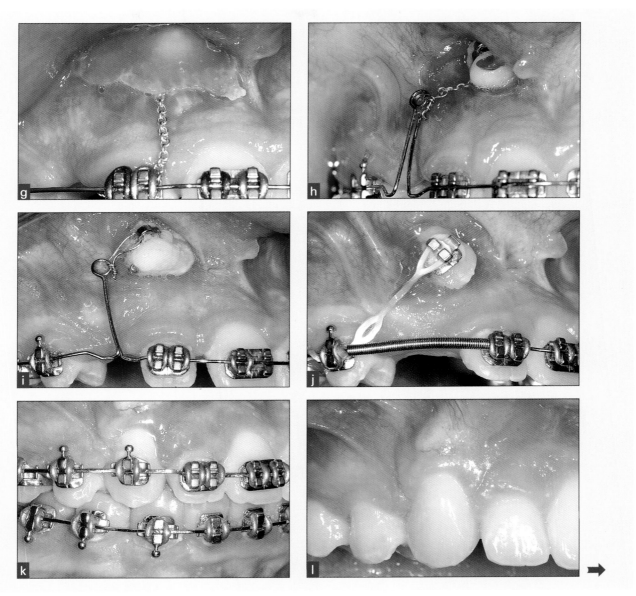

**(g)** A Barricaid dressing (Midwest Dental) was placed over the crown. **(h)** To avoid further damage to the root of the lateral incisor and to facilitate eruption of the canine, a labial force was applied to the tooth using a Ballista spring. **(i to k)** After the tooth had erupted sufficiently toward the labial, an elastomeric chain was used to gradually move the tooth into the dental arch. **(l and m)** After appliance removal, there was a discrepancy between the crown length of the right canine and the other maxillary anterior teeth.

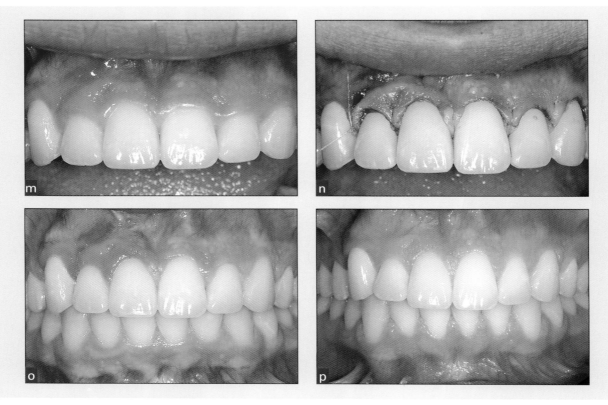

**(n)** Maxillary anterior crown lengthening was performed to improve the overall tooth proportions. **(o)** The final tooth position after appliance removal. **(p)** This tooth position was reasonably stable 5 years after the completion of treatment. (Orthodontics courtesy of Dr Vince Kokich, Jr, Tacoma, Washington.)

Before any surgery is initiated, it is imperative to determine the location of the impacted tooth. In the case of a labial impaction, the tooth may be palpable, and a bulge can be seen. However, it may be positioned in the middle of the alveolus or palatally, in which case it will not be palpable. In both situations, it will be necessary to determine its location by taking two radiographs at different angles. The buccal object rule[14]—when two different radiographs are made of a pair of objects, the image of the buccal object moves, relative to the image of the lingual object, in the same direction that the x-ray beam is directed—is helpful in determining the location of these impacted teeth. In Fig 2-6b, it was determined that the tooth was impacted labially, near the midalveolar region. It was ectopically positioned, and an APF was necessary to uncover and move it.

Occasionally, it is difficult to diagnose the exact location of impacted teeth when they are in the midalveolar region. Cone beam computed tomography (CBCT) imaging is very helpful in making the correct diagnosis to determine if the impacted tooth is on the labial or palatal of the roots of the adjacent teeth (see Fig 2-12).

## Ectopic labial impaction

The most common location for the ectopic labial impaction is mesial to the lateral incisor. Ideally, to use the APF on this type of impaction, there should be a minimum of 4 to 6 mm of gingiva on the adjacent central and lateral incisors. The authors prefer to sound the labial of the donor site to be sure the bone is at the normal level. If the bone is at a normal level, then a full-thickness flap can be employed. If there is a labial dehiscence, then a split-thickness flap should be used. At least a 2-mm width of gingiva should be incorporated with the pedicle flap. It is important to leave a 2- to 3-mm gingival collar around the incisor donor site (see Fig 2-2). Bone is removed from the crown of the impacted tooth, leaving an opening that is larger than the crown (see Fig 2-12). The flap is sutured to the periosteum with resorbable gut sutures, exposing the crown of the tooth. If there is concern that the tissue will re-cover the tooth quickly, then a bracket is bonded to the tooth and a dressing placed (see Fig 2-12). Orthodontic movement can be initiated in 6 weeks. This technique must be planned and performed very carefully. The impacted canine may be located directly over the root of the incisor, and a significant bony dehiscence may be present on the lateral incisor.

Presently, a modified flap design is being tested to uncover these ectopically impacted labial canines (Janakievski J, personal communication, 2013) (Fig 2-7). A horizontal incision is made from the central incisor to the premolar, just coronal to the mucogingival junction, so that it includes one to two millimeters of gingiva. The flap is elevated without using vertical incisions. Adequate access is achieved with this design so that bone can be removed from the crown of the canine with good visibility. The flap is apically positioned with resorbable sutures, leaving the crown of the canine uncovered. A bracket is bonded to the canine, and a dressing is placed over the surgical site. This technique can be employed prior to placement of orthodontic appliances. The author (DPM) has found that, similar to the preorthodontic uncovering technique for palatal canines, the canine will begin to erupt spontaneously (see Fig 2-7g). In addition, there is a wide border of attached gingiva after the tooth is orthodontically moved into position (see Fig 2-7h).

If there is inadequate gingiva over the incisor donor site, then the edentulous area could be considered for the pedicle flap (see Fig 2-8). This complicates the flap design because of the distance from the edentulous area to the impacted tooth. The surgery must be carefully planned to allow proper exposure of the impacted tooth and leave adequate gingiva over the central and lateral incisors. On very rare occasions, the impacted tooth will be so high up in the vestibule that flap access may be difficult or injudicious. In these cases, a simple window in the mucosa to access and uncover the tooth may be all that is possible (see Fig 2-12). Future gingival grafting or connective tissue grafting may be necessary after the tooth is in position. Occasionally, these impactions are so high and deep in the vestibule that uncovering and orthodontic movement is fraught with too many complications and risks. In this situation, extraction should be considered (see Fig 2-13).

## Fig 2-7 ) Spontaneous eruption of an impacted maxillary left canine after uncovering.

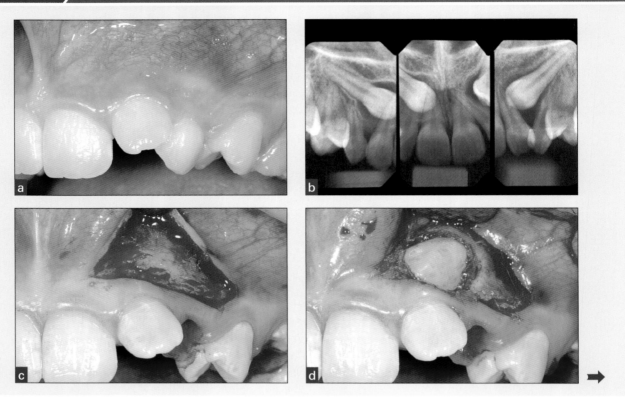

*(a)* The maxillary left canine in this adolescent girl was ectopically impacted and was lying on the root of the lateral incisor. *(b)* Using the buccal object rule,* the radiographs show that the maxillary left canine is labially impacted and ectopically positioned over the root of the lateral incisor. *(c)* A modified APF was elevated using a horizontal incision from the left central incisor to the first premolar. *(d)* Bone was removed from the crown of the impacted canine.

*When two different radiographs are made of a pair of objects, the image of the buccal object moves, relative to the image of the lingual object, in the same direction that the x-ray beam is directed.

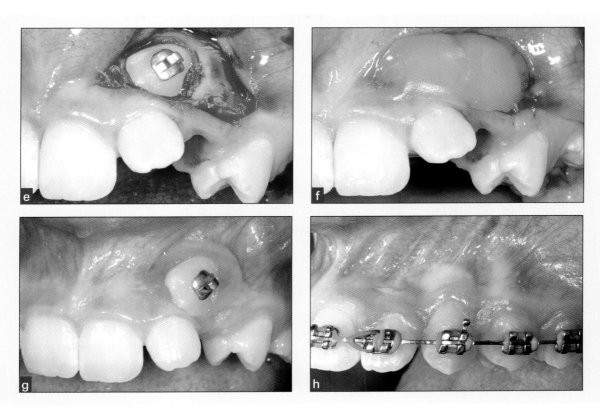

(*e and f*) A bracket was bonded to the impacted canine, and a Barricaid dressing was placed over the surgical area to keep the tooth uncovered. (*g*) Four months later, further spontaneous eruption had occurred. (*h*) Brackets were placed, and the tooth was erupted into its ideal position 16 months after the initial surgery. (Courtesy of Dr Doug Knight [orthodontist], and Dr Jim Janakievski [periodontist], Tacoma, Washington.)

## Labial, coronal, nondisplaced impaction

When the tip of the labially impacted tooth is coronal to the adjacent cementoenamel junction (CEJ) and there is a wide zone of attached gingiva, it may be possible to use the gingivectomy technique to uncover the crown of the impacted canine (see Fig 2-1). In this patient, a simple gingivectomy was possible. Two-thirds of the crown of the tooth was exposed, and no bone removal was necessary. After the gingivectomy, there was adequate remaining attached tissue. A dressing can be placed over the enamel to prevent tissue overgrowth. The dressing may be removed in 1 week. The patient is then instructed to keep the exposed crown clean with a toothbrush or a chlorhexidine rinse on a cotton swab to prevent gingival proliferation. In 3 weeks, the tissue will be healed sufficiently to allow the orthodontist to place a bracket and begin tooth movement. If this technique is used properly, there should be adequate attached gingiva and no recession when the orthodontic treatment is completed (see Figs 2-1g and 2-1h).

## Labial, apical, nondisplaced impaction

If the tip of the labially impacted canine is near the adjacent CEJ or slightly apical to it, then the APF or closed eruption technique should be used. In this location, it would be impossible to perform an excisional gingivectomy and leave an adequate zone of attached gingiva (see Fig 2-3).

The angle of the impaction will dictate which technique is best to use. If the tooth is tipped 30 to 45 degrees (see Fig 2-2), it may be difficult to extricate with the closed eruption technique. Consultation with the orthodontist will help in the decision as to which technique should be used in these borderline cases. The authors prefer to use the closed eruption technique whenever possible. In Fig 2-3, a closed eruption technique could have been used in lieu of the APF.

In the example shown in Fig 2-8, a split-thickness pedicle flap was reflected from the crest of the edentulous area, preserving as much gingiva as possible. The incisions were extended vertically into the vestibule, and the split-thickness flap was reflected. Occasionally, a thin shell of bone covers the enamel. This bone can be removed with a curette or surgical round bur, exposing the crown. The flap is sutured to the periosteum with resorbable sutures, leaving two-thirds of the crown exposed. If there is concern that tissue will proliferate over the tooth, a bracket and dressing can be placed. Orthodontic therapy can be initiated 6 weeks after the surgery.

If the tooth is vertically positioned with minimal angulation and impacted high in the vestibule or within the alveolus (midalveolar), then the closed eruption technique is the treatment of choice (see Fig 2-4).

## Fig 2-8 ) Horizontally impacted maxillary right canine.

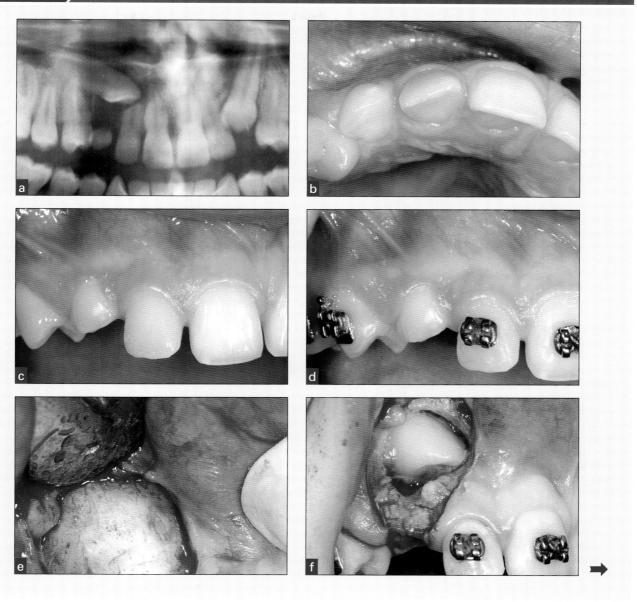

**(a and b)** The maxillary right canine in this adolescent girl was impacted horizontally and positioned slightly labial to and near the apex of the lateral incisor, tipping the tooth facially. **(c and d)** The maxillary primary canine remained in the dental arch during initial bracketing and alignment. **(e and f)** The primary canine was extracted, a pedicle flap was reflected, and bone was removed, uncovering two-thirds of the crown of the canine.

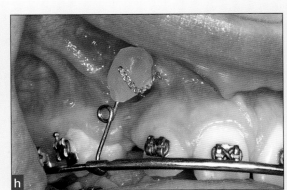
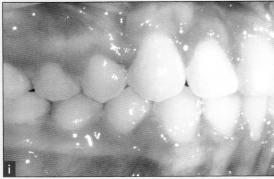
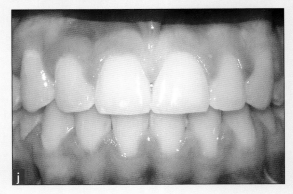

*(g)* A bracket and chain were bonded to the labial surface of the canine, and the flap was positioned apically. *(h)* Eight weeks later, a labial arch, extending from the maxillary left first molar to the maxillary right first molar, was used to anchor a spring that delivered a labial force to the canine crown. This facially directed force prevented further resorption of the lateral incisor root. *(i and j)* The posttreatment photographs show that the gingival levels of the canines and lateral incisors are identical to those on the contralateral side. (Orthodontics courtesy of Dr Tim Quinn, Gig Harbor, Washington.)

### Labial, midalveolar, high, nondisplaced impaction

The closed eruption technique is the treatment of choice in this situation (see Fig 2-5). A crestal incision can be made, and vertical incisions can help release the flap on the labial aspect. If the tooth is in the midalveolar location, it is helpful to make a sulcular incision on the palatal aspect of the adjacent teeth for better access. In this situation, the tip of the tooth is located and enough bone is removed to allow the widest part of the crown to pass though the access hole created in the bone (see Fig 2-4). If the tooth is labially displaced, there may be a thin shell of bone covering the crown. This is easily removed with curettes or round burs, exposing the crown. The tooth is isolated, cleaned, dried, and etched, and a bonding agent is placed. A chain is then bonded directly to the labial aspect of the tooth. If the tooth is in the midalveolar position, the chain can be bonded to the incisal edge. The flaps are returned to their original location for closure and sutured with resorbable sutures. The chain passes under the flap and exits at the midcrestal incision area, where it is attached to the archwire or adjacent bracket (see Fig 2-5). The orthodontist can activate force in 2 to 3 weeks. If proper mechanics are used, the tooth will erupt, as it would have naturally, through the crest of the ridge.

# Orthodontic Mechanics

The orthodontic mechanics to erupt a labially impacted canine should be directed appropriately to avoid damaging the roots and surrounding bone of the adjacent teeth and to facilitate physiologic movement of the impacted tooth. If the orthodontic mechanics are directed inappropriately, then the tooth movement may cease, root resorption could occur, and the labial bone support of the adjacent teeth could be in jeopardy. The position of the crown of the impacted tooth relative to the adjacent teeth and alveolar bone will dictate which type of mechanics are the most appropriate.

## Midalveolar impaction

If the impacted canine is positioned between the roots of the lateral incisor and first premolar, then it is likely in a midalveolar position, with intact labial and palatal plates of cortical bone covering the crown. In this situation, it is best not to remove extensive labial bone during the surgical procedure. These teeth are typically uncovered with the closed eruption technique. The surgeon will attach a chain to the crown that extends into the oral cavity through an opening in the crest of the alveolar ridge.

Although various types of mechanics can be employed to erupt the tooth vertically toward the maxillary occlusal plane, the authors' favorite is a Ballista loop constructed from 0.018-inch round archwire (see Figs 2-2 and 2-5). The length of the loop should be equal to the distance from the labial archwire to the center of the alveolar ridge (see Fig 2-2f). When the Ballista loop is not activated, it extends occlusally toward the opposite arch. When activated by rotating the loop apically and attaching it to the chain on the crown of the impacted canine, the force on the tooth is directly occlusally, and the tooth should erupt into the center of the ridge. This is important, because this type of eruption direction will have the least negative impact on the labial bone over the root.

When erupting the impacted tooth with a Ballista spring, it is possible to erupt the tooth too rapidly, because it is simply being pulled vertically and does not require any bone resorption to facilitate the movement. The authors recommend erupting an impacted tooth about 1 mm per month.

A mistake that is often made when erupting a midalveolar impaction is use of a chain to move the tooth in a labial direction. This can cause a dehiscence in the labial bone, which could lead to gingival recession. Therefore, occlusally directed mechanics will provide the least destructive path of movement.

Occasionally, if there is insufficient labial gingiva over a midalveolar canine impaction, it is necessary to perform an APF to uncover the tooth. In this situation, because the crown of the tooth is visible, a bracket can be placed on the tooth. Therefore, the mechanics to erupt the tooth could be simplified, and an elastomeric chain can be used to move the crown of the tooth occlusally (see Fig 2-3).

## Ectopic labial impaction

Most ectopic maxillary labial canine impactions are positioned mesially and over the root of the lateral incisor. As mentioned earlier in this chapter, the method of uncovering ectopic labial canines is to use an APF to permit access to and direct visualization of the canine crown. However, the mechanics to erupt a mesially positioned maxillary canine will depend on how high the canine is positioned relative to the root of the lateral incisor.

## Fig 2-9 ) Impacted maxillary left canine erupted with a bracket and chain.

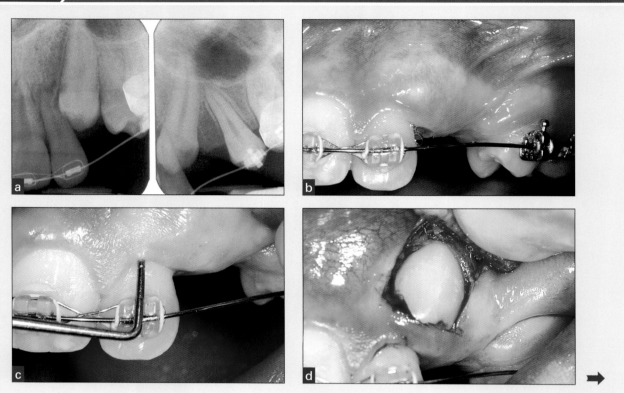

(a) The maxillary and mandibular first premolars were extracted to make space for the remaining teeth and to encourage the eruption of the maxillary left canine. (b) However, the canine did not erupt spontaneously. (c) The labial surface of the lateral incisor was sounded to plan the surgical approach. (d) A pedicle flap was reflected, leaving a wide collar of gingiva around the lateral incisor.

In some situations, the canine crown may be located at or near the midroot level of the adjacent lateral incisor (Fig 2-9; see also Fig 2-2). In these cases, after crown uncovering with an APF, about two-thirds of the canine crown will usually be positioned far enough to the labial so that a direct distal force from an elastomeric chain can be applied to move the tooth into the dental arch (see Fig 2-9). Because the crown is positioned outside of the alveolus, the enamel is not pushing against the bone as the tooth is being pulled distally. In these types of cases, the root is moving through the bone in a physiologic manner.

Figures 2-5 and 2-9 illustrate borderline cases in which the closed eruption technique could have been used. The tooth was angled less than 30 degrees, and closed orthodontic mechanics could have erupted this tooth. Again, consultation with the orthodontist will help in the decision making prior to the surgery.

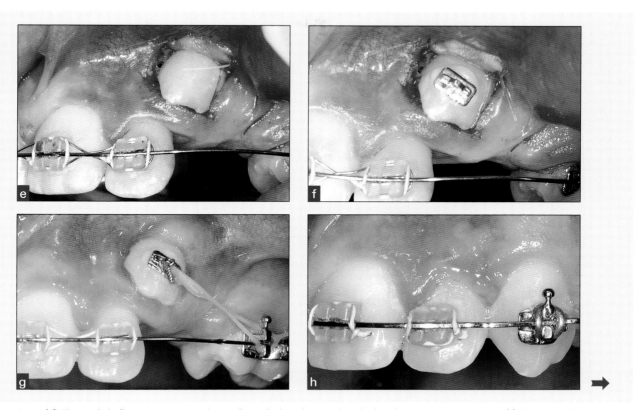

**(e and f)** The pedicle flap was positioned apically, and a bracket was bonded to the canine crown. **(g and h)** Eight weeks later, an elastomeric chain was used to erupt the canine into the dental arch.

In some cases (see Fig 2-2), to avoid damage to the lateral incisor root during distal movement of the canine crown, it is advantageous to move the source of the anchorage for the elastomeric chain more apically, using an additional archwire extension, so that the pull on the impacted crown is directly toward the distal and not occlusally oriented (see Fig 2-2). Once the direct distal force has moved the impacted crown past the underlying lateral incisor, a direct vertical pull with either the orthodontic archwire or an elastomeric chain can be used to erupt the tooth into position. In these types of cases, the bracket often must be removed from the lateral incisor while the canine crown is being moved distally. This allows the lateral root to move away if the canine crown comes too close during the retraction movement of the canine. This will avoid potential bone and root resorption on the lateral incisor.

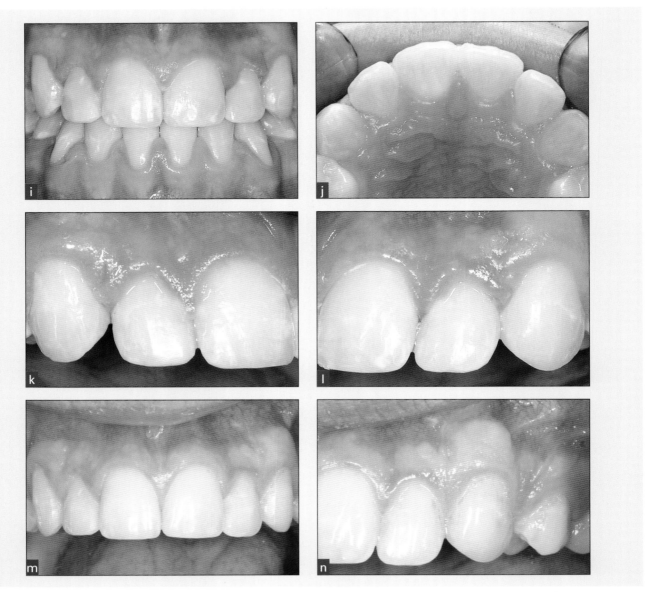

(*i to l*) The posttreatment photographs show that the gingival levels of the lateral incisor and previously impacted canine are nearly identical to those of the contralateral teeth. (*m and n*) Nine years after orthodontics, the tooth positions and tissue levels have remained stable.

## Fig 2-10  Transposed and labially impacted maxillary right canine.

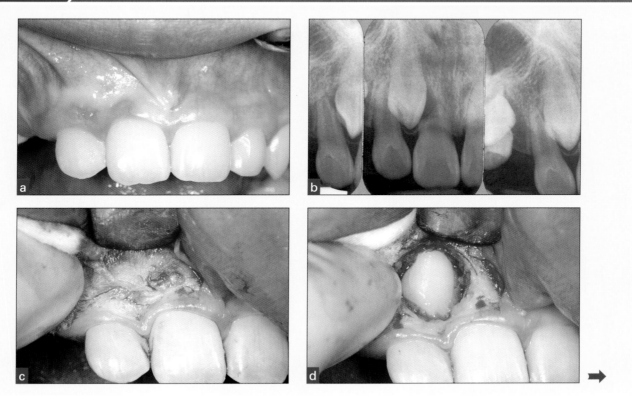

(*a and b*) The maxillary right canine in this adolescent girl was transposed and impacted labially between the roots of the maxillary right central and lateral incisors. It had already caused extensive root resorption of both the central and lateral incisors. (*c*) A split-thickness labial pedicle flap was reflected, leaving a collar of gingiva around the right central and lateral incisors. (*d*) The labial bone was removed, uncovering about two-thirds of the canine crown.

## Challenges

The greatest orthodontic challenges are the labial impactions that are positioned high and apically, very near the apex of the lateral incisor root. In these situations, the crown of the tooth is positioned deeper within the alveolus but still labial to the adjacent lateral incisor root apex. The most appropriate initial direction of movement for these teeth is directly labially (Figs 2-10 and 2-11; see also Figs 2-6 and 2-8). There are several different types of orthodontic appliance designs that can produce a direct labial movement. One option is to bend a Ballista loop into a 0.018-inch round archwire so that the unactivated loop is directed labially. Then when the loop is drawn up to the attachment on the canine, the force produced on the crown of the canine is toward the labial (see Figs 2-6h and 2-6i). After the crown of the tooth has been moved far enough labially, an elastomeric chain can be used to move the tooth distally and occlusally (see Figs 2-6j and 2-6k).

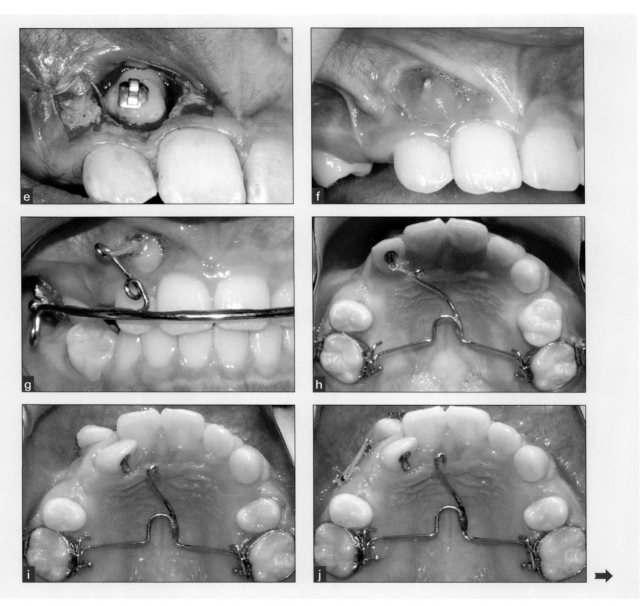

**(e and f)** A cleat was bonded to the tooth, the pedicle flap was apically positioned and sutured, leaving the crown exposed, and a Barricaid dressing was placed over the crown. **(g)** Six weeks after surgery, orthodontic traction of the canine was initiated. To avoid further damage to the central and lateral incisor roots, a 0.045-inch labial bow was attached to both maxillary first molars, and an auxiliary loop was placed on the bow to deliver a labially directed force to the impacted canine. **(h)** In addition, a palatally directed force was placed on the lateral incisor to move it away from the canine. **(i to k)** After the canine crown had moved labially and the lateral incisor had moved palatally, a miniscrew was placed mesial to the maxillary right second premolar to anchor an elastomeric chain, which was used to gradually retract the right canine.

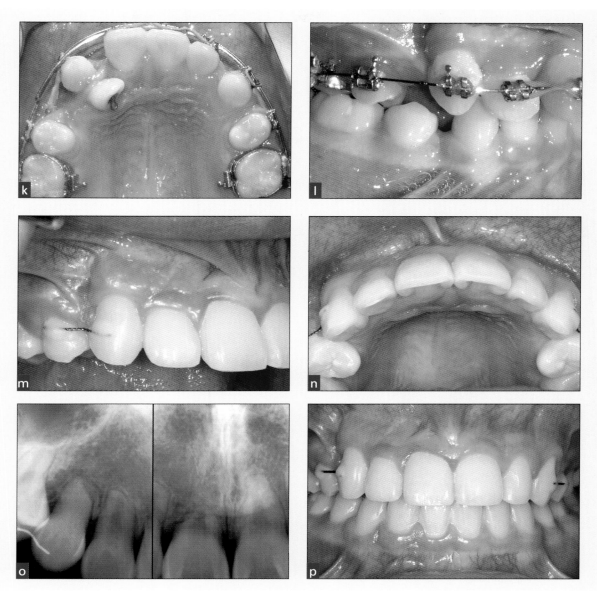

(l) Eventually, brackets were placed on the maxillary teeth to complete the alignment of the lateral incisor and canine. (m and n) After bracket removal, a flexible wire was bonded to the right canine and second premolar to help prevent relapse of space closure. (o) Although the patient had short roots at the end of the treatment, there has been minimal resorption from the initial radiograph. (p) The 4-year posttreatment photograph shows that the tooth position has been stable and the esthetic appearance of the teeth is excellent. (Orthodontics courtesy of Dr Tim Quinn, Gig Harbor, Washington.)

**Fig 2-11** ) **Impacted maxillary left canine causing extensive root resorption.**

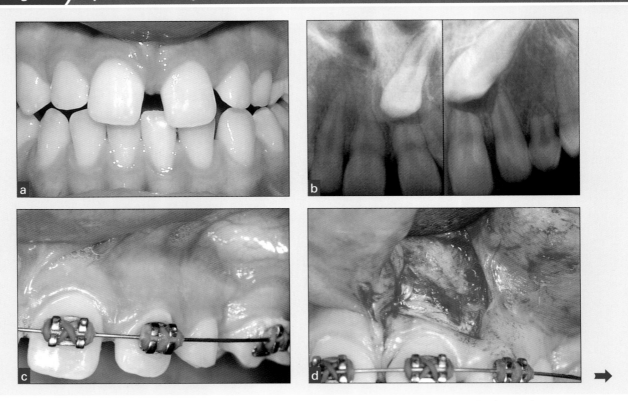

*(a and b)* The maxillary left canine in this adolescent girl was impacted in the midalveolar region and had caused extensive resorption of the roots of the central and lateral incisors. *(c)* Brackets were placed to obtain initial tooth alignment. The buccal object rule and direct palpation were used to determine that a labial approach was appropriate to uncover the crown. *(d)* A pedicle flap was reflected from the central incisor, leaving a collar of gingiva around the central incisor.

The mistake that is often made by the orthodontist is to attempt to move a deeply impacted labial canine directly toward the distal with the initial movement. This does not produce a physiologic type of tooth movement. When the enamel of the impacted crown is pulled distally against the adjacent alveolar cortical bone, pressure is created and, for a while, nothing happens, because enamel has no way of resorbing the bone except through pressure necrosis. Eventually, the bone will give way, but this process can take an inordinate amount of time and can cause reciprocal movement of the anchor teeth toward the slowly moving impacted canine.

Another method of moving a deeply impacted maxillary canine in a directly labial direction is to use an auxiliary labial bow that attaches into the headgear tubes of the maxillary first molars and extends between these anchor teeth. A vertical wire can be soldered to this labial bow (see Figs 2-8 and 2-9). The soldered auxiliary wire should extend to the height of the labial impaction. A loop can be placed in the soldered auxiliary wire to deliver a direct labial force on the tooth so that it will move immediately out of the alveolus and can then be directed in a distal direction. An elastomeric chain can also be attached from the crown of the impacted canine to the auxiliary wire to create the force necessary to move the crown out of the bone.

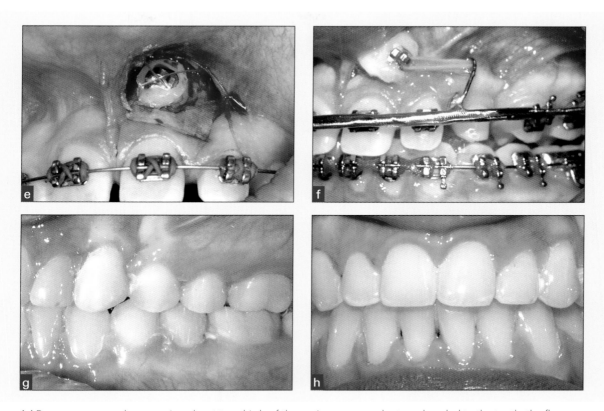

*(e)* Bone was removed, uncovering about two-thirds of the canine crown, a cleat was bonded to the tooth, the flap was apically positioned to leave the crown exposed, and the primary canine was extracted. *(f)* A 0.045-inch labial bow with an auxiliary spring was used to deliver a labially and distally directed force to avoid further damage to the incisor roots. *(g and h)* The posttreatment photographs show that the canine was successfully positioned into occlusion with an ideal esthetic appearance of the maxillary anterior teeth. (Orthodontics courtesy of Dr Tim Quinn, Gig Harbor, Washington.)

The position of the adjacent lateral incisor can be an impediment to the efficient movement of the labially and ectopically impacted maxillary canine. In some situations, therefore, it is actually better to move the lateral incisor into the palate initially (see Fig 2-10), using a palatal bar with an auxiliary wire that can be used to move the lateral incisor palatally. After the canine has been moved sufficiently distally so that the lateral incisor root will not be injured, the lateral incisor can be moved back into its normal position in the dental arch (see Fig 2-10).

Occasionally, a labial and ectopic canine will be impacted over the root of the maxillary central incisor (see Fig 2-11). In these situations, it is absolutely imperative that the canine crown be moved out toward the labial before the orthodontic force is directed distally. If an orthodontist makes the mistake of moving the tooth in a directly distal direction, it not only could jeopardize the root of the central and lateral incisors but also could severely affect the bone levels of these teeth after the orthodontic treatment has been completed. After the crown is moved significantly labial and away from the central incisor (see Fig 2-11), it can be gradually moved distally and eventually into the dental arch.

## Attaching to the tooth

The simplest and best attachment to use with the closed eruption technique is to bond the chain directly to the tooth without using a bracket (see Fig 2-5). This is more secure and less obtrusive. When the tissue is repositioned over the tooth, there is less likelihood that a perforation will occur over the chain. A bracket, being more obtrusive, may perforate the tissue and cause a gingival defect requiring gingival or connective tissue grafting.

# Important Considerations

### Imaging

Many clinicians request CBCT images of their labial canine impaction cases in order to document the exact position of the canine crown prior to surgical uncovering. Because CBCT scans permit a three-dimensional (3D) appraisal of the canine and adjacent lateral and central incisors,[15-21] it is possible to view the degree of labial root resorption that exists with many of these lateral incisors prior to orthodontic treatment (Fig 2-12). In fact, it is frightening to see that the resorption often encroaches on the pulp canal of the lateral and central incisors. These teeth are often so severely compromised by the labial root resorption that they should be considered to have significantly guarded prognoses. However, for many years, 3D imaging was not available, so we never realized the extent of the labial root resorption that was present. That being said, the authors have not seen the loss of a lateral incisor or central incisor due to labial root resorption in any of their patients over the past 35 years. Previous studies have shown that labial resorption routinely heals itself by deposition of secondary cellular cementum over the exposed dentin.[22,23] In addition, seldom do these teeth require root canal therapy.

## Fig 2-12 ) Labially impacted maxillary left canine near the apex of the lateral incisor.

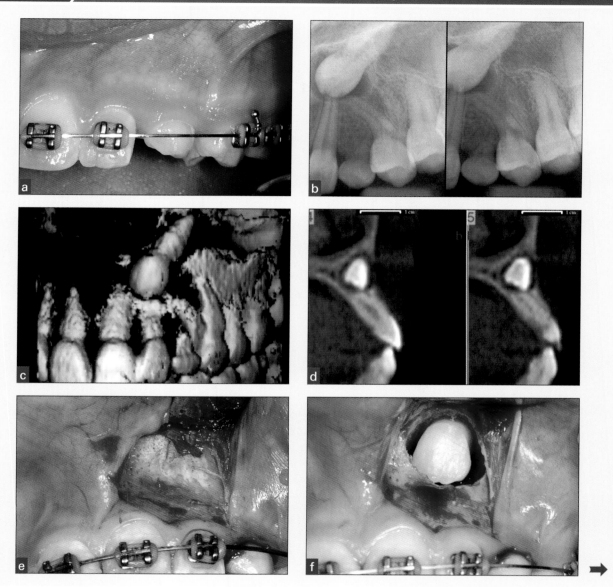

*(a and b)* The maxillary left canine was impacted labially and near the apex of the root of the lateral incisor. *(c and d)* The surface-rendered image as well as the multiplanar sections reproduced from a CBCT scan show that the crown of the impacted canine is positioned slightly to the labial of the lateral incisor root apex. *(e)* A full-thickness pedicle flap was reflected, preserving a collar of gingiva around the central and lateral incisors. *(f)* Bone was removed, exposing the crown of the impacted canine.

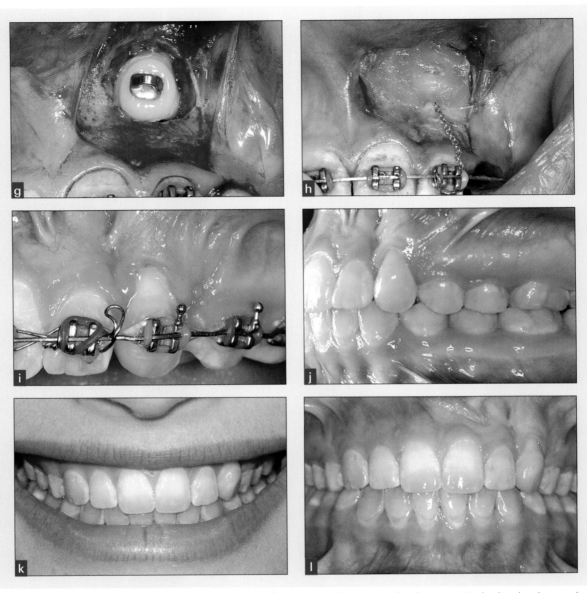

(*g and h*) A cleat was bonded to the canine crown, the flap was apically positioned, a chain was attached to the cleat, and a Barricaid periodontal dressing was placed over the exposed tooth. (*i*) The tooth was erupted into the dental arch, and some recession was noted, which would be treated later with a connective tissue graft. (*j to l*) Final orthodontic finishing. (Orthodontics courtesy of Dr Roy Gunsolus, Seattle, Washington.)

## Esthetics

Vermette et al[24] compared the periodontal and esthetic results of patients treated with closed eruption and APF techniques and found no significant differences in gingival index, plaque index, pocket depth, and bone level between the two. However, they identified significant esthetic differences between these two uncovering techniques. With an APF, the crown length of the impacted tooth is longer than normal because of apical migration of the gingival margin (see Fig 2-6m). The crown lengths of teeth uncovered with the closed eruption technique were similar to their contralateral nonimpacted counterparts. In addition, high labial impactions uncovered with an APF tend to reintrude after orthodontic treatment because of the healing of the APF to the mucosa adjacent to the impacted tooth at the time of uncovering. As the tooth erupts into the dental arch, the mucosa is drawn coronally. After orthodontic treatment, this mucosal attachment tends to pull the crown of the tooth apically. This disadvantage was not observed in teeth uncovered with closed eruption. Becker et al[25] found similar favorable esthetic results in their study of the closed eruption technique for uncovering impacted maxillary central incisors.

## Gingival recession

Problems are sometimes encountered when labially impacted canines are ectopically located. These teeth need to be left uncovered with the APF technique. The orthodontist must use an extrusive labial force to initiate movement to "jump" the impacted canine over the lateral incisor (see Fig 2-10). There is a greater tendency for gingival recession on those teeth that are very displaced and are very apically positioned (see Fig 2-12). In the authors' experience, these teeth usually have inherent dehiscences before treatment is initiated. If the patient has a thin phenotype, there is a higher incidence of recession. These patients are easily treated with a connective tissue graft after orthodontic treatment is completed. Total root coverage is often accomplished with this treatment (see Fig 4-4).

Prophylactic treatment with a gingival graft can be performed to reduce the risk of labial recession on the lateral incisor (see Fig 2-2). In this particular case, a pedicle was reflected from the lateral incisor, leaving a very narrow band of gingiva. The canine was ectopically positioned labial to the lateral incisor, and tooth movement across the lateral incisor could have caused recession, so adequate width was established by grafting the lateral incisor to prevent this from occurring.

## Lack of tooth movement

The authors have encountered a few cases in which the closed eruption technique was improperly used and the chain was entrapped with new bone formation after flap closure[26] (see Fig 7-11c). When a surgeon elevates a flap to expose a high labial impaction, the typical procedure is to perform a full mucoperiosteal flap elevation. However, if the surgeon then attaches a chain to the impacted crown, lays that chain against the denuded bone, and covers the bone and chain with the flap, the periosteum will be covering the chain. The internal layer of the periosteum consists of osteoblasts, so the periosteum will begin to deposit bone beneath the cellular layer and eventually entrap the chain in bone. Of course, an orthodontist would be unable to move the tooth and could presume that it is ankylosed. This is a surgical mistake.

The solution to this problem would be to elevate a split-thickness flap near the alveolar crest, allowing the periosteum to remain over the crestal alveolar bone. Then a full-thickness flap is elevated over the impacted tooth to allow for attachment of the chain or anchoring device. When the chain is then laid down prior to flap replacement, the chain will be outside of the periosteum and there will be no risk of bone entrapping the chain.

## Root resorption

Some of the patients illustrated in this chapter demonstrated preorthodontic root resorption of the adjacent lateral incisor and often the central incisor (see Figs 2-5 to 2-8 and 2-10 to 2-12). Previous authors have also documented varying degrees of root resorption following the treatment of maxillary labial canine impactions.[27–33] In some cases, the resorption was significant and the loss of root length was substantial. Although the exact cause and effect of the root resorption are not well substantiated, we assume that the encroaching follicle of the ectopically erupting canine comes into close proximity with the lateral incisor root. In most cases, the lateral root will autonomously move away from the canine crown as it erupts. However, in some situations, the lateral incisor and central incisor roots do not move and begin to resorb. When significant loss of root length is present, the canine crown is located within the alveolus or midalveolar region.

The authors have followed several of these patients for many years after treatment and have observed that the root resorption always ceases after the orthodontic treatment. This observation has been documented by Remington et al[34] in a large series of orthodontic patients with moderate to severe root resorption that were evaluated more than 10 years after removal of orthodontic appliances.

It is important for general dentists and pediatric dentists to monitor the eruption of the maxillary canines on panoramic and periapical radiographs during the mixed dentition (ie, ages 7 to 11). During this time, the proximity of the canine relative to the adjacent lateral incisor and central incisor roots should be assessed.[35] If it is noted that an adjacent developing canine is encroaching on the lateral incisor root and causing some initial resorption, it may be wise to extract the primary canine on that side to encourage the developing canine to change its path of eruption and assume a more normal eruptive path. If, on subsequent radiographs, the resorption of the lateral incisor is still proceeding and the canine path of eruption has not been altered, then the authors recommend uncovering the canine and beginning an initial phase of orthodontic treatment immediately, before all permanent teeth have erupted, to move the canine labially and stop the root resorption of the lateral incisor. Complete orthodontic treatment can be delayed until the remaining permanent teeth have erupted, but at least the root resorption of the lateral incisor will have been stopped, enhancing the future prognosis of this tooth.

## Direction of tooth movement

Some surgeons recommend "troughing" of the bone adjacent to an ectopic labially impacted maxillary canine.[36] The theory is that removing the bone will provide less resistance to the canine crown as it moves distally through the alveolar ridge. However, the authors do not recommend troughing of the alveolus, believing that the ideal physiologic process is to move the root, not the crown, through the bone. Therefore, in cases where the canine crown is submerged within the alveolus, the authors always move the crown labially as a first step. Then, once the crown is labial to the adjacent alveolar cortical bone, the crown is moved distally toward its eventual position in the dental arch. During the distal movement, the root moves through the bone, so the process occurs in a more physiologic rather than a destructive manner. Excessive bone removal from troughing could cause a problem with future bone support of the canine after orthodontic correction. Additionally, if for some reason the canine cannot be moved into its site and extraction is necessary, preservation of bone is imperative for a future implant. Therefore, the authors do not recommend the troughing procedure.

## Crown length discrepancies

Occasionally, there will be a discrepancy in gingival levels after the orthodontic treatment is completed. This can be due to recession on the impacted tooth or a short clinical crown on the contralateral canine (see Fig 2-6) and is more common in the case of the high labially impacted tooth. If this is an esthetic problem, it can be corrected with either a gingivectomy or osseous surgery on the contralateral canine or a connective tissue graft on the previously impacted canine. If the contralateral canine is the problem, the appropriate technique will be dictated by the bone level and amount of gingiva on the tooth. Usually, osseous surgery is needed because the bone is close to the CEJ and the normal biologic width (approximately 2 mm from the CEJ) needs to be established. Conservative flap reflection and osseous contouring will correct this problem and make the canines equal in length (see Fig 2-6). If there is adequate attached gingiva and excessive sulcular depth (3 to 4 mm), a simple gingivectomy can be done (see Fig 2-1).

Interestingly, when the closed eruption technique is used, the crown length may be too short when the case is completed (see Fig 2-4). This occurs because the tooth was in the middle of the alveolus and no labial bony dehiscence was present. This is easily corrected with the aforementioned techniques.

## Lateral incisor positioning

A consequence of ectopic eruption and labial impaction of a maxillary canine is that the root of the lateral incisor tends to become displaced lingually (see Fig 2-10). As a result, the crown of the lateral incisor is often proclined labially. During initial orthodontic therapy, it is best not to attach the archwire to the lateral incisor until the canine has been moved away from the lateral incisor root. When the lateral incisor is attached to the archwire, correction of the root angulation is a slow process. Ectopic labially impacted canine cases always require extra time during orthodontic finishing to correct the angulation of the lateral incisor roots. This is accomplished by using a large-sized rectangular archwire with labial root torque placed into the wire to move the root labially and the crown palatally. In some situations, it is advantageous to also use auxiliary torquing springs to facilitate this type of tooth movement. One of the risks with torquing the lateral root is that additional root resorption could occur as the root is moved labially. Therefore, in those patients with extensive lateral incisor root resorption due to an impinging ectopically erupting canine, it may be necessary to compromise the final lateral incisor root position in favor of avoiding additional root resorption.

## Fig 2-13  Impacted maxillary canines requiring extraction of permanent teeth.

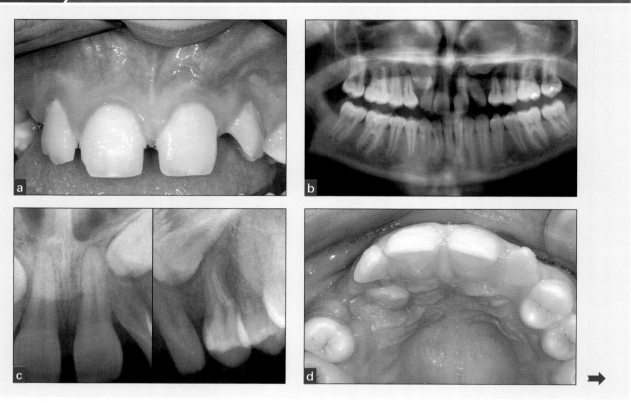

**(a to d)** Both maxillary canines were impacted in this adolescent girl. The right canine was positioned palatally and was uncovered and allowed to erupt autonomously. The left canine was positioned above the root apices of the left central and lateral incisors. There was a significant arch length discrepancy in the maxillary arch, which required extraction of permanent teeth.

## Extraction versus movement

There are occasions in which it is more prudent to extract the labially impacted maxillary canine rather than correct its position.[37–41] In these cases, there should be an accompanying arch length deficiency in the maxillary arch and a satisfactory facial profile to warrant the extraction of maxillary first premolars (Fig 2-13). However, if the first premolar is well positioned in the dental arch, then it may not make good sense to extract the premolar and then go through a difficult orthodontic repositioning of the impacted canine. The more prudent decision may be to extract the impacted canine and to substitute the first premolar for the canine in the final occlusal scheme.

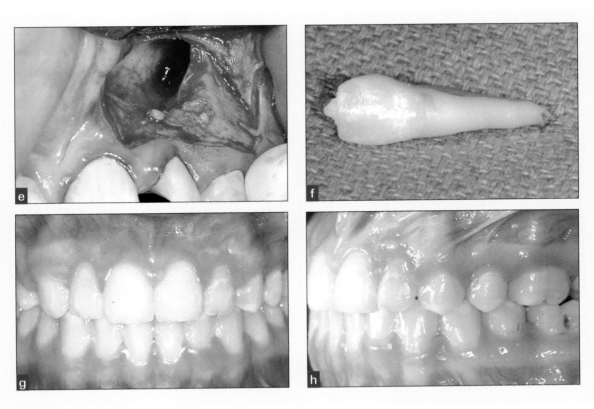

(*e and f*) The maxillary right first premolar and maxillary left canine were extracted to create space for the remaining teeth. (*g and h*) In the final occlusal scheme, the maxillary left first premolar was substituted for the maxillary left canine. (Orthodontics courtesy of Dr Doug Knight, Tacoma, Washington.)

# References

1. Bass T. Observations on the misplaced upper canine tooth. Dent Pract 1967;18:25–33.

2. Johnston WD. Treatment of palatally impacted canine teeth. Am J Orthod 1969;56:589–596.

3. Chung DD, Weisberg M, Pagala M. Incidence and effects of genetic factors on canine impaction in an isolated Jewish population. Am J Orthod Dentofacial Orthop 2011;139:331–335.

4. Sajnani AK, King NM. The sequential hypothesis of impaction of maxillary canine: A hypothesis based on clinical and radiographic findings. J Craniomaxillofac Surg 2012;40:375–385.

5. Kim Y, Hyun HK, Jang KT. Interrelationship between the position of impacted maxillary canines and the morphology of the maxilla. Am J Orthod Dentofacial Orthop 2012;141:556–562.

6. Yan B, Sun Z, Fields H, Wang L, Luo L. Etiologic factors for buccal and palatal maxillary canine impaction: A perspective based on cone-beam computed tomography analyses. Am J Orthod Dentofacial Orthop 2013;143:527–534.

7. Williams B. Diagnosis and prevention of maxillary cuspid impaction. Angle Orthod 1981;51:30–40.

8. Bonetti A, Parenti I, Zanarini M, Marini I. Double vs single primary teeth extraction approach as prevention of permanent maxillary canines ectopic eruption. Pediatr Dent 2010;32:407–412.

9. Olive RJ. Orthodontic treatment of palatally impacted maxillary canines. Aust Orthod J 2002;18:64–70.

10. O'Neill J. Maxillary expansion as an interceptive treatment for impacted canines. Evid Based Dent 2010;11:86–87.

11. Vanarsdall R, Corn H. Soft tissue management of labially positioned unerupted teeth. Am J Orthod 1977;72:53–64.

12. Kokich V, Mathews D. Surgical-orthodontic management of impacted teeth. Dent Clin North Am 1993;37:181–204.

13. Kokich VG. Surgical and orthodontic management of impacted maxillary canines. Am J Orthod Dentofacial Orthop 2004;126:278–283.

14. Richards A. The buccal object rule. Dent Radiogr Photog 1980;122:9–14.

15. Haney E, Gansky S, Lee J, et al. Comparative analysis of traditional radiographs and cone-beam computed tomography volumetric images in the diagnosis and treatment planning of maxillary impacted canines. Am J Orthod Dentofacial Orthop 2010;137:590–597.

16. Algerban A, Jacobs R, Fieuws S, Willems G. Comparison of two cone beam computed tomographic systems versus panoramic imaging for localization of impacted maxillary canines and detection of root resorption. Eur J Orthod 2011;33:93–102.

17. Botticelli S, Verna C, Cattaneo P, Heidmann J, Melsen B. Two- versus three-dimensional imaging in subjects with unerupted maxillary canines. Eur J Orthod 2011;33:344–349.

18. Wriedt S, Jaklin J, Al-Nawas B, Wehrbein H. Impacted upper canines: Examination and treatment proposal based on 3D versus 2D diagnosis. J Orofac Orthop 2012;73:28–40.

19. Rossini G, Cavallini C, Cassetta M, Galluccio G, Barbato E. Localization of impacted maxillary canines using cone beam computed tomography. Review of the literature. Ann Stomatol (Roma) 2012;3:14–18.

20. Jung Y, Liang H, Benson B, Flint D, Cho B. The assessment of impacted maxillary canine position with panoramic radiography and cone beam CT. Dentomaxillofac Radiol 2012;41:356–360.

21. Sajnani A, King N. Diagnosis and localization of impacted maxillary canines: Comparison of methods [epub ahead of print 14 December 2012]. J Investig Clin Dent doi:10.1111/j.2041-1626.2012.00163.x.

22. Ericson S, Kurol J. Incisor root resorptions due to ectopic maxillary canines imaged by computerized tomography: A comparative study in extracted teeth. Angle Orthod 2000;70:276–283.

23. Owman-Moll P, Kurol J, Lundgren D. Repair of orthodontically induced root resorption in adolescents. Angle Orthod 1995;65:403–408.

24. Vermette M, Kokich V, Kennedy D. Uncovering labially impacted teeth: Closed eruption and apically positioned flap techniques. Angle Orthod 1995;65:23–32.

25. Becker A, Brin I, Ben-Bassat Y, Zilberman Y, Chaushu S. Closed-eruption surgical technique for impacted maxillary incisors: A postorthodontic periodontal evaluation. Am J Orthod Dentofacial Orthop 2002;122:9–14.

26. Bonetti A, Incerti Parenti S, Daprile G, Montevecchi M. Failure after closed traction of an unerupted maxillary permanent canine: Diagnosis and treatment planning. Am J Orthod Dentofacial Orthop 2011;140:121–125.

27. Falahat B, Ericson S, Mak D'Amico R, Bjerklin K. Incisor root resorption due to ectopic maxillary canines: A long-term radiographic follow-up. Angle Orthod 2008;78:778–785.

28. Algerban A, Jacobs R, Lambrechts P, Loozen G, Willems G. Root resorption of the maxillary lateral incisor caused by impacted canine: A literature review. Clin Oral Investig 2009;13:247–255.

29. Brusveen E, Brudvik P, Boe O, Mavragani M. Apical root resorption of incisors after orthodontic treatment of impacted maxillary canines: A radiographic study. Am J Orthod Dentofacial Orthop 2012;141:427–435.

30. Kim Y, Hyun H, Jang K. The position of maxillary canine impactions and the influenced factors to adjacent root resorption in the Korean population. Eur J Orthod 2012;34:302–306.

31. Lai C, Bornstein M, Mock L, Heuberger B, Dietrich T, Katsaros C. Impacted maxillary canines and root resorptions of neighbouring teeth: A radiographic analysis using cone-beam computed tomography. Eur J Orthod 2013;35:529–538.

32. Yan B, Sun Z, Fields H, Wang L. Maxillary canine impaction increases root resorption risk of adjacent teeth: A problem of physical proximity. Am J Orthod Dentofacial Orthop 2012;142:750–757.

33. Strbac GD, Foltin A, Gahleitner A, Bantleon H, Watzek G, Bernhart T. The prevalence of root resorption of maxillary incisors caused by impacted maxillary canines. Clin Oral Investig 2013;17:553–564.

34. Remington D, Joondeph D, Artun J, Riedel R, Chapko M. Long-term evaluation of root resorption occurring during orthodontic treatment. Am J Orthod Dentofacial Orthop 1989;96:43–46.

35. Garib DG, Janson G, Baldo T, Dos Santos P. Complications of misdiagnosis of maxillary canine ectopic eruption. Am J Orthod Dentofacial Orthop 2012;142:256–263.

36. Crescini A, Baccetti T, Rotundo R, Mancini E, Prato G. Tunnel technique for the treatment of impacted mandibular canines. Int J Periodontics Restorative Dent 2009;29:213–218.

37. Garcia B, Boronat A, Larrazabal C, Penarrocha M. Immediate implants after the removal of maxillary impacted canines: A clinical series of nine patients. Int J Oral Maxillofac Implants 2009;245:348–352.

38. Patel S, Fanshawe T, Bister D, Cobourne M. Survival and success of maxillary canine autotransplantation: A retrospective investigation. Eur J Orthod 2011;33:298–304.

39. De Oliveira M, Pithon M. Attempted traction of impacted and ankylosed maxillary canines. Am J Orthod Dentofacial Orthop 2012;142:106–114.

40. Boffano P, Schellino E, Giunta G, Gallesio C. Surgical removal of impacted maxillary canines. J Craniofac Surg 2012;23:1577–1578.

41. Mirabella D, Giunta G, Lombardo L. Substitution of impacted canines by maxillary first premolars: A valid alternative to traditional orthodontic treatment. Am J Orthod Dentofacial Orthop 2013;143:125–133.

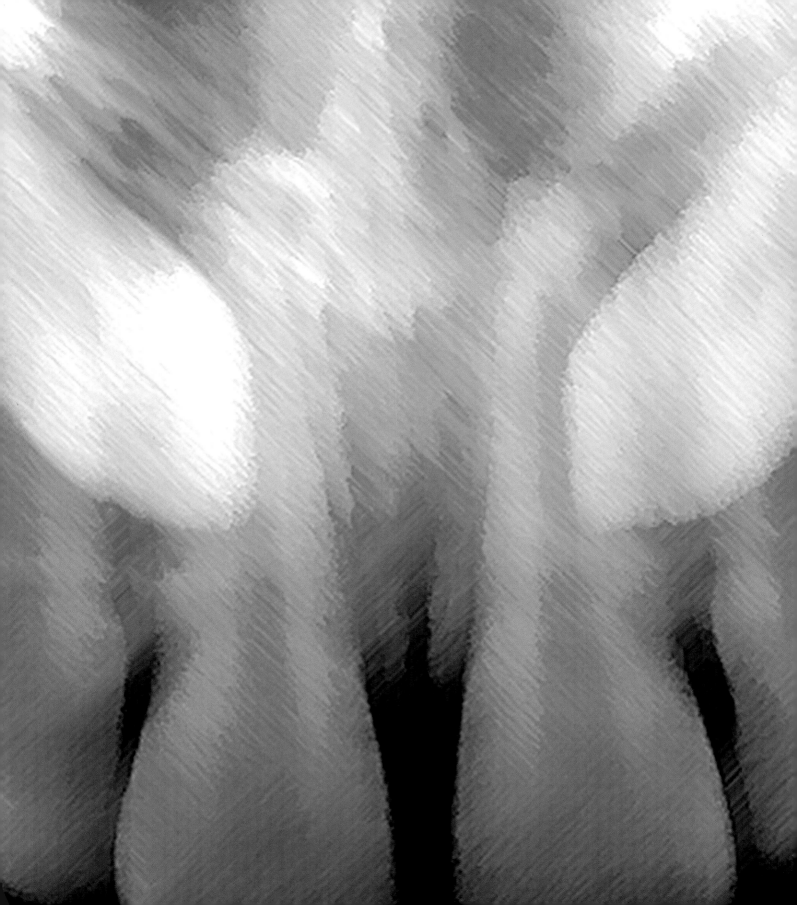

# Palatally Impacted Canines ( 3 )

As mentioned in the previous chapter, maxillary canines are the second most commonly impacted teeth, after mandibular third molars.[1] While one-third of canines are labially impacted, two-thirds are palatally impacted.[2-4] It is estimated that palatal canine impaction affects between 1.0% and 2.5% of the general population.[5,6] In addition, there are radiographic predictors of consequences of palatally impacted canines.[7-10] Palatal canine impaction can be managed by either preventive (interceptive) or surgical treatment.

## Interceptive Treatment

Sometimes extraction of the primary canine can be an effective way to facilitate the eruption of the impacted canine, as long as the impaction is diagnosed at a young age and the crown of the impacted canine does not lie past the root of the adjacent lateral incisor.[11-13] However, primary canine extraction will be ineffective when the impacted tooth is positioned too far toward the mesial. This is more likely to occur if the diagnosis is made at a later age.[6]

In addition, there is another preventive method that can be employed to erupt palatally impacted canines. Ectopically positioned maxillary canines can be erupted by extracting the primary canine and then opening space orthodontically between the maxillary lateral incisor and the primary first molar or permanent first premolar, depending on the dentition of the patient.[14–17] This orthodontic space opening will allow the impacted canine to erupt toward the center of the alveolar ridge. However, the forcing apart of the lateral incisor and first molar will often require further treatment to close any remaining gaps between teeth.

Leonardi et al[18] reported that the application of cervical headgear in addition to maxillary primary canine extraction in young adolescents improved eruption pathways of palatally impacted permanent canines in 80% of patients. However, because cervical headgear is specific to certain types of orthodontic treatment, this technique cannot be used across the board for all patients with palatally impacted canines.

Most referrals for palatal canine impaction do not occur until the patient's teeth are fully erupted or the canine crown is positioned mesially past the lateral incisor root. In such cases, surgical exposure of the canine is the only effective treatment, followed by orthodontic movement of the tooth into the dental arch.[19] If the crown of the palatally impacted canine is uncovered surgically, the tooth can erupt either autonomously or through guided orthodontic eruption. The following sections discuss the differences between these two surgical approaches to palatal canine impaction.

## Closed Eruption Surgical Technique

The closed eruption technique (Fig 3-1) involves the elevation of a mucoperiosteal flap, exposure of the palatally impacted canine crown, removal of sufficient bone to allow tooth movement, attachment of a gold chain (which will exit through the palatal flap), and repositioning of the flap to re-cover the tooth (see Fig 3-1g). The tooth can be orthodontically guided into the dental arch after the area has healed. For many years, the closed eruption technique has been used successfully to erupt palatally impacted canines. However, the eruption process can cause root resorption of the adjacent lateral incisor, bone loss, and adverse periodontal effects.

Becker and Zilberman,[20] in their study of the proper eruption pathway for palatally impacted canines using the closed eruption technique, concluded that the eruptive force should be directed lingually and away from the root of the lateral incisor. This force direction avoids canine-to–palatal bone contact and would therefore prevent root damage to the lateral incisor. After the crown erupts into the oral cavity, it can be orthodontically moved to the proper canine position.

Many orthodontists simply pull the tooth laterally toward the edentulous ridge instead of erupting the impacted canine distally and palatally away from the adjacent central and lateral incisors. This often causes the canine crown to compress against the adjacent palatal bone. The enamel of the crown cannot resorb the adjacent bone physiologically, so this crown-to-bone contact leads to pressure necrosis, which will result in bone resorption as the impacted canine moves laterally. In addition, no bone remodeling occurs behind the canine crown as the advancing crown erupts.

# Fig 3-1 ) Palatally impacted maxillary canines near the nasopalatine foramen.

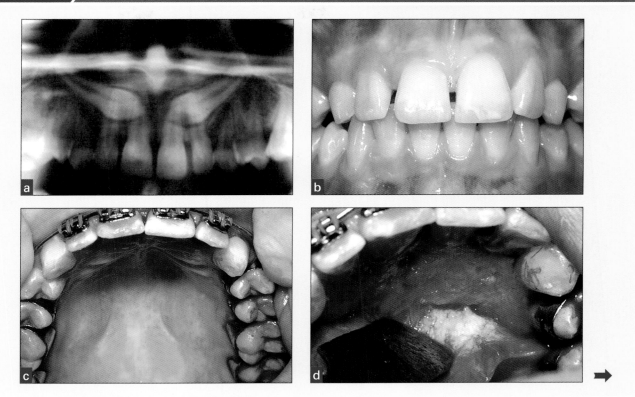

(a) This adolescent girl had two palatally impacted maxillary canines that were nearly approximating one another near the nasopalatine foramen. (b) She had an Angle Class I malocclusion with spacing in the maxillary anterior region. (c) Brackets and bands were initially placed on all teeth, and the dental arches were aligned. (d) A full-thickness palatal flap was reflected from the maxillary right premolar to the maxillary left premolar. Both canines were completely covered with bone.

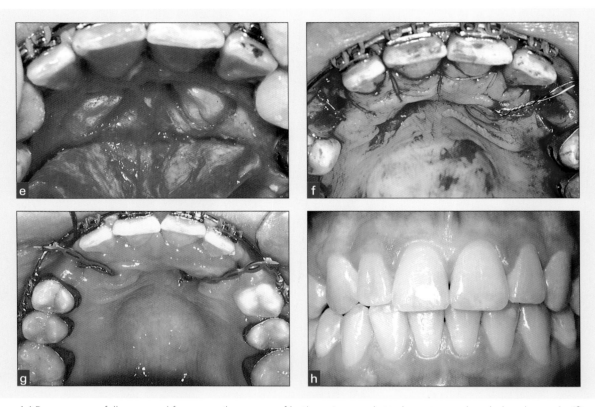

(*e*) Bone was carefully removed from over the crowns of both canines, and attachments were bonded to the teeth. (*f*) Ligating wires were attached to the brackets, and the flap was fenestrated and repositioned with resorbable sutures. The ligating wire passed through the fenestration and was attached to the archwire. (*g*) Six weeks postoperatively, elastomeric chains were attached from the canines to the archwires to move the teeth laterally. (*h*) After the completion of orthodontic treatment, the canines have been moved into their proper position within the maxillary arch.

This type of forced movement has been shown to result in bone levels and attachment levels on the distal of the lateral incisor and mesial of the previously impacted canine that are more apical than the contralateral lateral incisor and nonimpacted canine.[21–27] Therefore, the esthetics are negatively impacted. However, the closed eruption technique does not have to result in bone resorption or poor attachment levels around the previously impacted canine. Therefore, the direction of eruption pathway of the canine crown beneath the palatal tissue is critical. For the most predictable outcomes with the closed eruption technique, the impacted tooth should first be erupted lingually and then moved laterally so as not to compromise the bone levels or cause root resorption of the lateral incisor (see Figs 3-8g, 3-9e, and 3-9f).

**Fig 3-2** Simple palatally impacted maxillary left canine exposed by soft tissue punch.

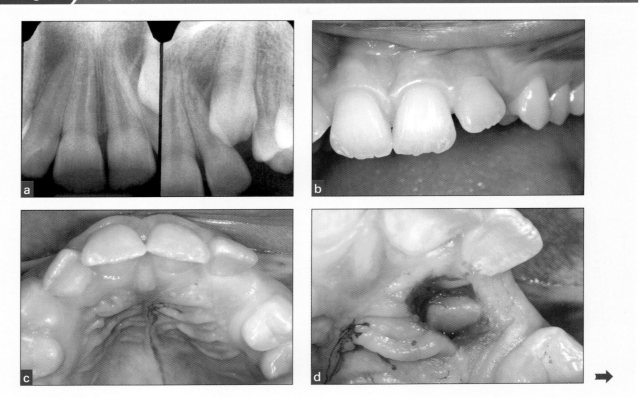

*(a)* This adolescent patient had an impacted maxillary left canine. Using the buccal object rule, one can deduce that the canine was impacted palatally. *(b and c)* The maxillary anterior teeth, including the contralateral canine, were completely erupted. A palatal prominence was evident in the region of the left canine crown, indicating that the tooth was located superficially. *(d)* Prior to the placement of orthodontic brackets, an excisional gingivectomy was performed to expose the crown of the canine. Bone removal was not necessary.

# Preorthodontic Uncovering Technique and Autonomous Eruption

Most impacted maxillary canines are located palatally. They are classified as *simple* impactions when they are not too deeply embedded within the alveolus (see Figs 3-2 to 3-4). They are classified as *complex* when they are deeply impacted and positioned near or above the apices of the roots of the maxillary lateral and central incisors (see Figs 3-5 to 3-8 and 3-10).

(e) A dressing was placed directly onto the crown of the tooth and was removed after 2 weeks. (f) Six months after uncovering, the orthodontic brackets were placed, the teeth were aligned, and sufficient space was created for the canine to erupt toward the edentulous ridge. (g) After the canine had erupted sufficiently, it was bracketed and aligned with the adjacent teeth. (h) The posttreatment photograph shows that the gingival margins of the nonimpacted and previously impacted maxillary canines are at the same level. (Orthodontics courtesy of Dr Doug Knight, Tacoma, Washington.)

## Simple palatal impactions

Simple palatal canine impactions are best treated by surgically uncovering the tooth and allowing it to erupt autonomously before beginning orthodontic treatment.[2,28,29] These teeth can be uncovered with a soft tissue punch technique or a flap. If the palatally impacted canine is coronally positioned and very superficial, a prominent palatal bulge can often be seen. A soft tissue punch procedure may be all that is needed to uncover the crown of the tooth (Fig 3-2). There is usually no bone covering these canines, so soft tissue removal may be all that is required. A dressing can be placed if there is concern about tissue overgrowth. When the canine is more deeply embedded and apically positioned, flap access facilitates the surgical uncovering (Fig 3-3).

## Fig 3-3 ) Palatally impacted maxillary right canine exposed by flap reflection.

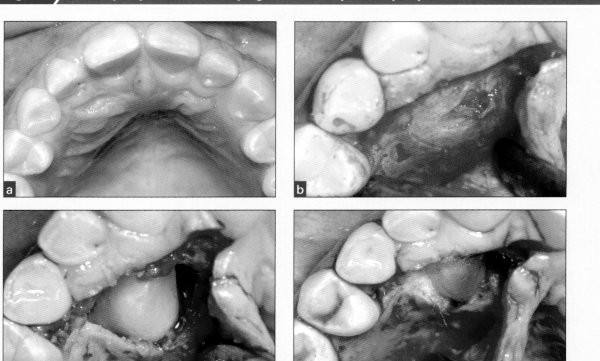

(a) This adolescent girl had a palatally impacted maxillary right canine. (b) A full-thickness palatal flap was reflected from the midline to the mesial of the first molar. A collar of gingiva was left around the central and lateral incisors. (c) Bone was removed, exposing the lingual surface of the impacted canine. (d) The tooth was isolated with Hemodent pledgets (Premier USA) for control of hemorrhage, and an etchant was placed on the lingual surface.

The uncovering technique requires flap reflection and complete bone removal from the coronal aspect of the tooth. If the primary canines are present, they are extracted at the time of the uncovering procedure. A full-thickness palatal flap is reflected from the premolar up to the midline (see Fig 3-3b). A 2- to 3-mm collar of gingiva can be left around the palatal of the lateral and central incisor. A curette or surgical round bur is used to locate the impacted tooth by gently removing the encasing bone (see Fig 3-3c). The crown of the tooth is exposed. Removal of the follicle around the periphery is not necessary and may increase the amount of bleeding during the procedure. This will complicate the surgery if bracket placement is necessary. At this point, experience will help in the decision to bond a bracket to help retain a dressing. If the tooth is not deeply embedded within the palatal bone and the surgeon feels that it will not re-cover with tissue during the healing process, then a bracket and dressing are not needed. Before flap closure, the area of the flap over the impacted tooth is scalloped, so that it leaves the tooth exposed after the flap is sutured (see Fig 3-3e).

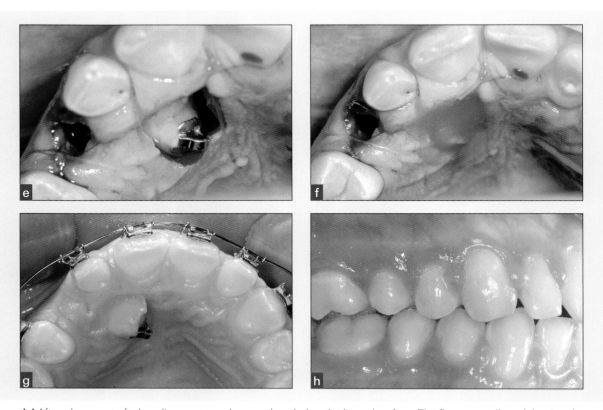

(**e**) After placement of a bonding agent, a cleat was bonded to the lingual surface. The flap was scalloped, leaving the cleat exposed. The primary canine was extracted at this time. (**f**) A light-cured dressing was attached to the cleat. (**g**) Four months later, the tooth had erupted vertically and distally away from the lateral incisor. (**h**) After the completion of orthodontics, the canine has been moved into its proper position relative to the adjacent teeth and opposing dental arch. (Figs 3-3a to 3-3c and 3-3e to 3-3g reprinted from Kokich[30] with permission.) (Orthodontics courtesy of Dr Doug Knight, Tacoma, Washington.)

If the tooth is more deeply embedded in the bone, a cleat is placed, which will retain a dressing more predictably. The flap is scalloped and sutured, and a light-cured peri-odontal dressing (Barricaid, Midwest Dental) is attached to the cleat (see Fig 3-3f). The dressing will ensure that the tissue does not re-cover the exposed tooth. This dressing can be left for up to 5 months if necessary (see Fig 3-10). During this time, the tooth, without orthodontic assistance, will start erupting above the surface of the palatal tissue. The dressing can then be removed. The other advantage of placing a bracket on these deeply embedded impactions is ease of re-uncovering if the dressing comes off prematurely and the healing tissue re-covers the tooth. It is a simple matter of a minor gingivectomy to uncover the bracketed tooth and place a new dressing or attach an orthodontic appliance.

In most cases, the tissue margins around the impacted tooth will epithelialize in 4 to 6 weeks (Figs 3-4 to 3-7).

### Fig 3-4 ) Palatally impacted maxillary left canine exposed via full-thickness flap.

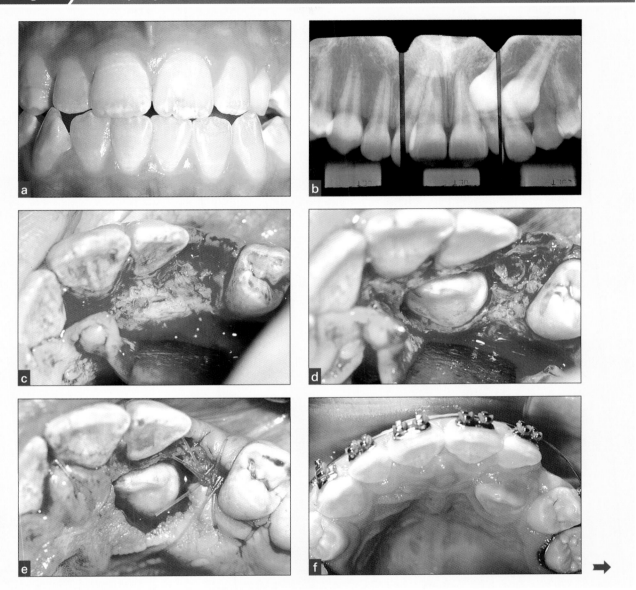

(a) This adolescent girl had a mild Angle Class III malocclusion with a reasonably balanced facial profile. As a result, her treatment required extraction of the mandibular right and left second premolars to establish an ideal anterior overjet. (b) In addition, the patient had an impacted maxillary left canine. Using the buccal object rule, one can ascertain that the canine was impacted palatally. (c) A full-thickness palatal flap was reflected from the first premolar to the left central incisor. The palatal bone was covering the canine crown. (d) This thin shell of bone was carefully removed with a curette and a round bur to expose the entire crown of the tooth. The marginal bone on the lingual of the central and lateral incisors was untouched. (e) The palatal flap was scalloped around the canine, repositioned, and sutured with resorbable sutures. (f) Six months after surgery, the canine had erupted significantly. Brackets were then placed on the maxillary teeth, and space was created for the canine.

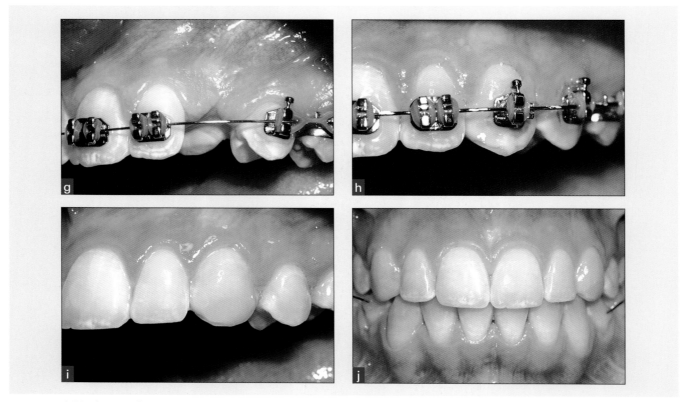

(g) By the time the maxillary teeth were aligned, the canine had erupted to the level of the occlusal plane of the maxillary dental arch. (h) The canine was then moved labially with orthodontic traction. (i and j) When one compares the gingival margins of the previously impacted left canine with the nonimpacted right canine, the levels are esthetic and identical.

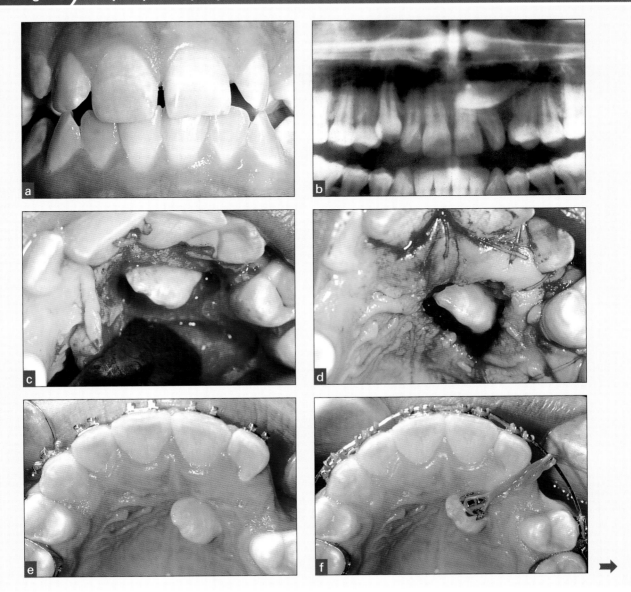

(a) This adolescent boy had an Angle Class I malocclusion with mild crowding in both dental arches. His orthodontic treatment did not require the extraction of any teeth. (b) The panoramic radiograph shows that his maxillary left canine was impacted horizontally at the level of the root apices of the maxillary left central and lateral incisors. (c) Prior to placement of orthodontic appliances, a full-thickness flap was elevated from the first premolar to the right central incisor. Bone was removed, exposing the crown of the canine. (d) The palatal flap was fenestrated and repositioned using resorbable sutures. No dressing was placed over the crown. (e) Six months postoperatively, the canine had erupted autonomously. Brackets were placed on the maxillary teeth, and space was created for the left canine. (f) An elastomeric chain was used to move the canine laterally toward the maxillary archwire.

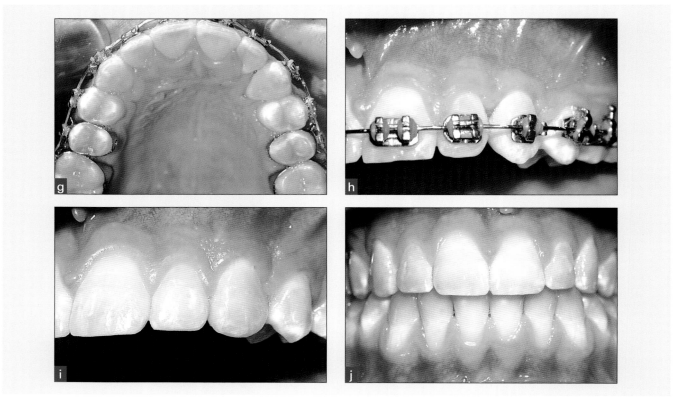

(**g and h**) After the crown had been moved into the dental arch, a rectangular archwire was used to torque the root labially. (**i and j**) After appliance removal, the gingival margins of the nonimpacted right canine and the previously impacted left canine are esthetic and identical.

## Fig 3-6 ) Palatally impacted maxillary canines exposed via full-thickness flap.

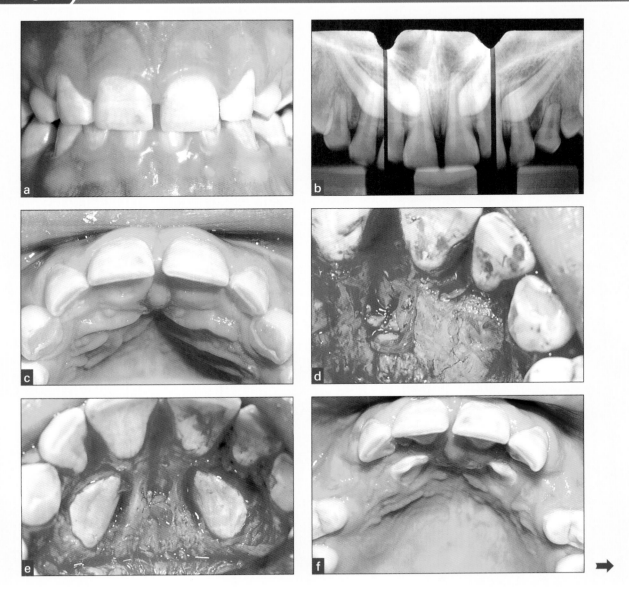

(a) This adolescent girl had an Angle Class I malocclusion with no arch length deficiency in either dental arch. (b) Both right and left maxillary canines were impacted palatally. (c) The prominences of the canine crowns are visible in the occlusal photograph. (d) A full-thickness flap was elevated and extended from the maxillary right to the left first premolars. Palatal bone was covering the canine crowns. (e) Bone was removed, exposing the entire crowns of the canines, and the flaps were fenestrated and repositioned. (f) Six months postoperatively, the orthodontics had not yet been started, but the canines had erupted autonomously about 5 mm.

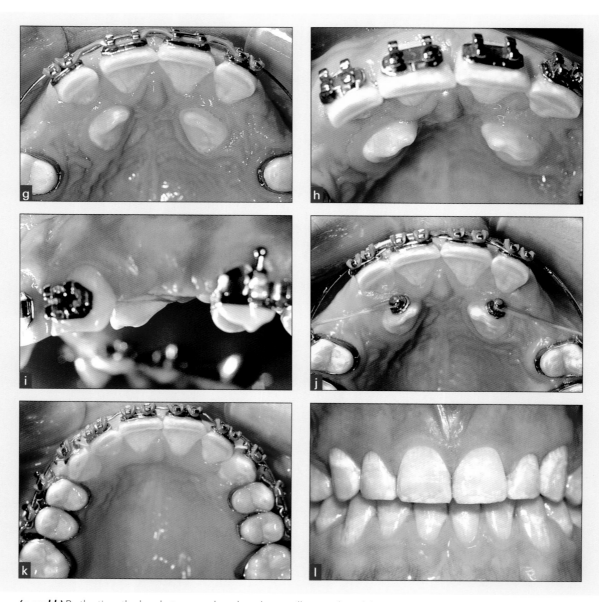

**(g and h)** By the time the brackets were placed on the maxillary teeth and the space was consolidated between the incisors, the canines had erupted even farther. **(i)** One year after uncovering (6 months after beginning orthodontics), the canines had erupted an additional 5 mm to the level of the maxillary occlusal plane. **(j and k)** Brackets were then bonded to the canines, and elastomeric chains were used to move the canines into alignment in the maxillary dental arch. **(l)** After orthodontic appliance removal, both canines have been positioned properly in the dental arch with the gingival margins at their appropriate esthetic levels relative to the incisors.

## Fig 3-7 ⟩ Palatally impacted maxillary canines exposed via separate full-thickness flaps.

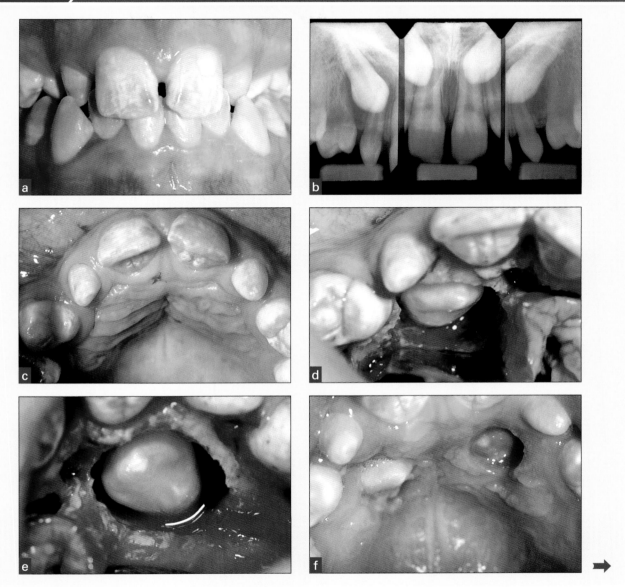

(a) This adolescent boy had an Angle Class I malocclusion with moderate crowding of both dental arches. However, his facial profile dictated a nonextraction orthodontic treatment plan. He had evidence of moderate fluorosis of all teeth. In addition, he had narrow, peg-shaped lateral incisors. (b) Using the buccal object rule, one could ascertain that both canines were impacted palatally. (c) The occlusal photograph shows the palatal prominences of the canine crowns. (d and e) Separate full-thickness flaps were elevated and extended from the first premolars to the incisive foramen. The bony coverings over the canines were removed, exposing the entire crown of each tooth. The flaps were fenestrated and repositioned with resorbable sutures. No dressing was placed. (f) Six months postoperatively, the canines had erupted autonomously a significant distance.

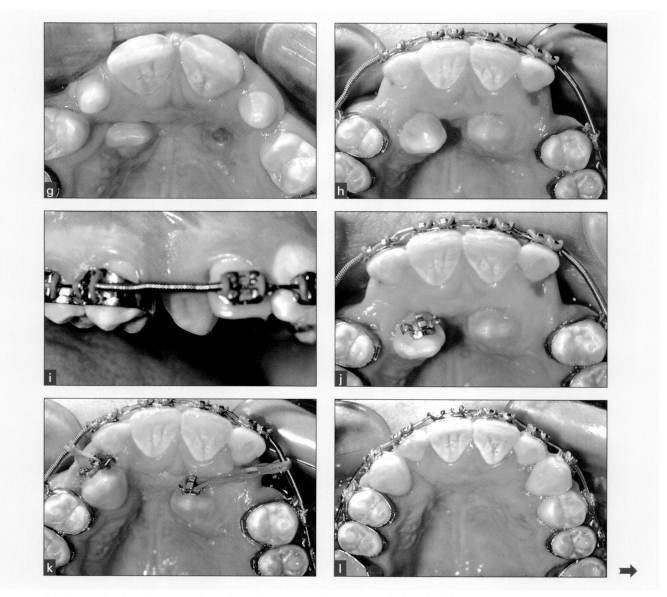

(g) Ten months after the surgery, the right canine was erupting more rapidly than the left canine. However, the orthodontic treatment was not started until both canines had erupted significantly. (h) The peg-shaped lateral incisors were built up with composite, brackets were placed on all the maxillary teeth, and space was created for the canine crowns. (i and j) The right canine erupted autonomously past the occlusal plane of the maxillary dental arch, so it was bracketed first, and an elastomeric chain was used to move it toward the archwire. (k and l) The left canine was also bracketed after it had erupted sufficiently, and both canines were eventually positioned properly in the maxillary dental arch.

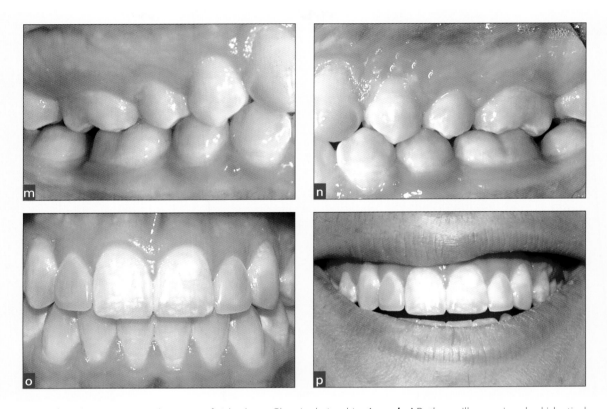

(m and n) The posterior occlusion was finished to a Class I relationship. (o and p) Both maxillary canines had identical gingival margins, which provided an esthetic smile for this adolescent boy. (Figs 3-7b, 3-7d, 3-7i, and 3-7o reprinted from Kokich[30] with permission.)

## Complex palatal impactions

It is uncommon to find a palatal impaction that cannot be treated with the preorthodontic uncovering technique. However, there are cases in which the canine is so deeply impacted and so apically positioned that a different approach should be considered.[31] These impactions are difficult to keep uncovered because of their depth. A full-thickness flap is reflected from the molar through the midline (Fig 3-8). Bone is removed from the crown of the impacted tooth, taking care not to damage the roots of the central incisor or lateral incisor, especially around the apices of these teeth. The area is isolated to achieve a dry field for bracketing. Surgical notes should be made of the tooth and its bone relationship. Documenting the surgery photographically will help the orthodontist in choosing the appropriate mechanics to erupt the tooth. A cleat is bonded to the tooth. A hemostat is used to grab the bracket to test the bond and verify that the tooth is mobile and not ankylosed.

If the tooth is ankylosed, it can be luxated to break it loose. However, it will most likely re-ankylose. Ankylosis is more common in the adult patient. In their 30 years of treating these impactions, the authors have never encountered an ankylosed palatal impaction in an adolescent. After the bond is tested, the flap is fenestrated with a #15 blade, so

**Fig 3-8** ) **Severely impacted maxillary right canine positioned above the apices of the incisors.**

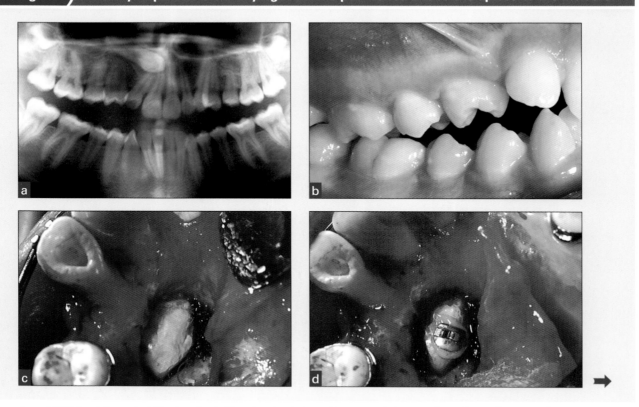

*(a and b)* This adolescent girl had an Angle Class I malocclusion with a severely impacted maxillary right canine that was positioned above the apices of the right central and lateral incisors. *(c)* A full-thickness flap was elevated, and the thick bony covering over the crown was removed to expose the crown of the canine. *(d)* A bracket was bonded to the palatal surface of the canine. The flap was fenestrated and repositioned with resorbable sutures.

that the bracket protrudes through the window in the flap (see Fig 3-8d). The palatal flap is returned to its original position and sutured with resorbable sutures using a continuous sling technique. A chain is attached to the cleat and runs outside the flap, where it attaches to the archwire. In 2 to 3 weeks, the orthodontist can initiate tooth movement. Appropriate mechanics must be applied to this very difficult impaction. A lingual transpalatal archwire will be needed to erupt a canine with this type of impaction using extrusive and distal force (see Figs 3-8e and 3-8f).

## Palatal impactions in adults

Preorthodontic uncovering of palatally impacted canines has also been performed in adults. The eruption process is much slower, but these canines will sometimes still erupt spontaneously when the overlying bone and tissue are removed. For adults over 30 years old, the authors recommend uncovering the palatally impacted canine and allowing it to erupt autonomously before applying force. It can then be erupted actively into the palate with a palatal spring and then moved laterally into the dental arch (Fig 3-9). Sometimes, however, the canine will not erupt and must be extracted.[32]

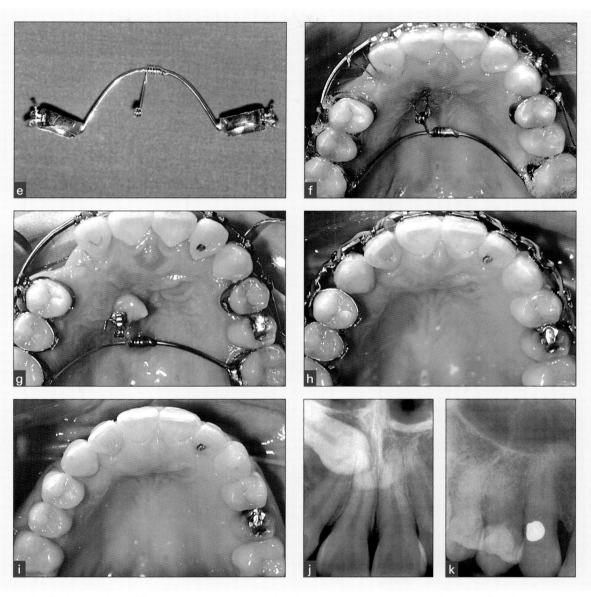

(e) A palatal arch with a soldered spring was constructed and cemented to the maxillary molars. (f and g) The spring was used to erupt the canine toward the center of the palate to avoid damaging the roots of the central and lateral incisors. (h and i) After the crown had been sufficiently erupted orthodontically, a bracket was bonded to the labial surface, the tooth was moved into the dental arch, and the orthodontic appliances were removed. The pretreatment (j) and posttreatment (k) periapical radiographs show the canine root position before and 20 years after completion of the orthodontic treatment. Note the dilacerated root of the right canine.

## Fig 3-9　Palatally impacted maxillary canines in a 41-year-old patient.

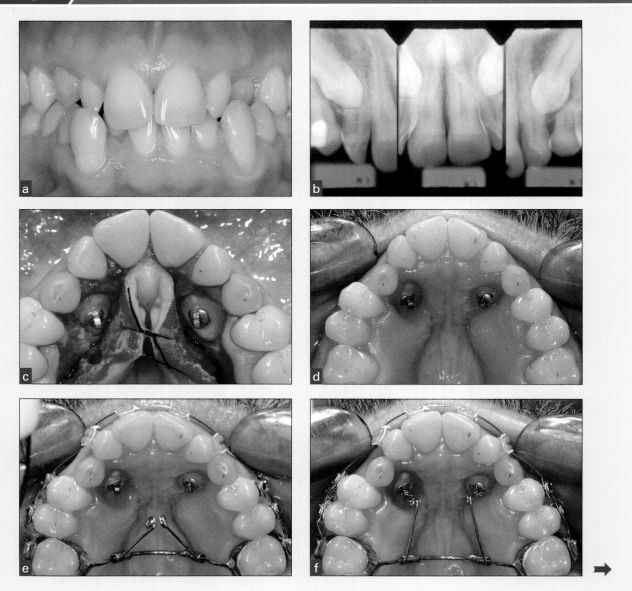

**(a)** This 41-year-old patient had an Angle Class I malocclusion with moderate mandibular incisor crowding, a narrow maxillary arch, maxillary lateral incisor crossbites, and palatal impaction of both maxillary canines. **(b)** Using the buccal object rule, one can determine from the pretreatment periapical radiographs that the canines are impacted palatally. **(c)** Prior to the placement of orthodontic appliances, full-thickness flaps were elevated, bone was removed from the crowns of the impacted teeth, and brackets were bonded to the lingual surfaces. The flaps were repositioned, the tissue was scalloped over the bracketed canines, and a dressing was placed. **(d and e)** Three weeks after the surgery, a palatal bar was constructed and cemented to the maxillary molars. Two erupting springs were soldered to the bar. **(f)** The springs were activated to deliver a palatally directed eruptive force on the canines. The primary canines were allowed to remain in the arch during this time for esthetic reasons.

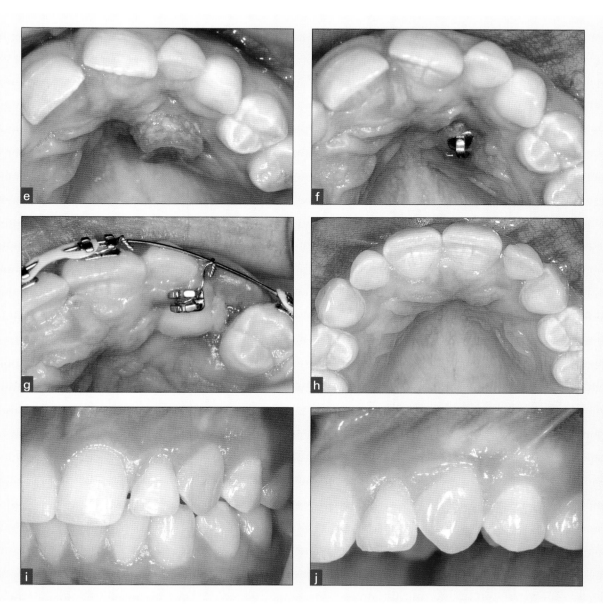

*(e and f)* The dressing remained on the crown for 5 months without replacement. When the tooth erupted to the surface of the palate, the long plug of dressing material was removed. The patient requested that the primary canine remain in the arch during these 5 months for esthetic reasons. *(g)* The orthodontic brackets were bonded to the teeth, and the canine was moved toward the dental arch. *(h to j)* Six years after the completion of orthodontics. (Orthodontics courtesy of Dr Steve Alexander, Olympia, Washington.)

**Fig 3-11** ) **Palatally impacted maxillary canines causing significant root resorption.**

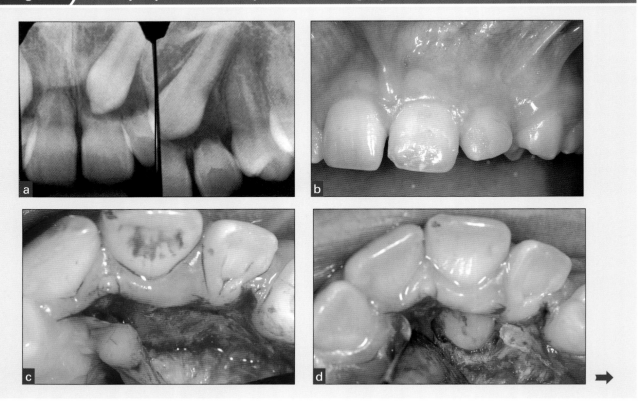

**(a)** This adolescent girl had two maxillary canines that were impacted in the midalveolus and had caused significant root resorption of all four maxillary incisors. **(b)** The patient had a moderate maxillary arch length deficiency that would require extraction of two teeth. The decision was made to extract the maxillary lateral incisors and eventually position the canines in the lateral incisor positions (two mandibular premolars would be extracted to preserve a Class I occlusion). **(c and d)** A full-thickness palatal flap was designed to leave a gingival collar on the lingual surface of the central incisor. Bone was carefully removed, exposing the impacted maxillary canine.

## Root resorption

Root resorption and bone loss of adjacent teeth can occur with improper orthodontic mechanics and improper timing of the tooth movement (Fig 3-11). These problems can be avoided when the tooth is properly uncovered and allowed to naturally erupt for months before initiating orthodontic mechanics.

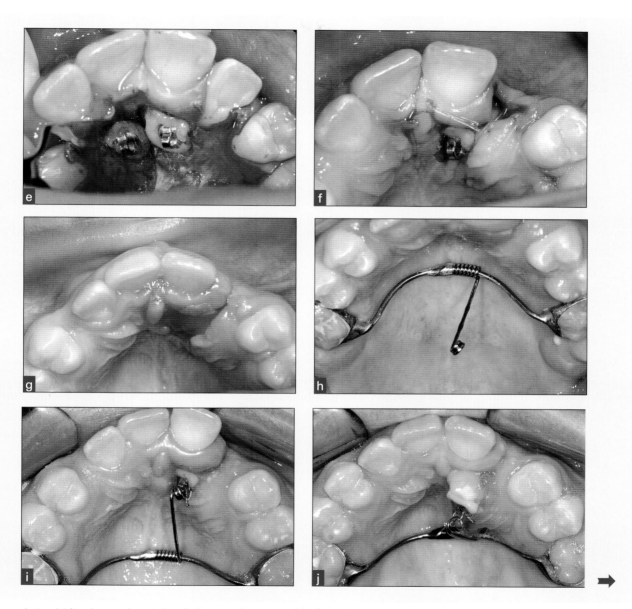

(*e to g*) A bracket was bonded to the impacted crown, and the lateral incisor was extracted. The flap was fenestrated and repositioned with resorbable sutures, and a dressing was attached to the bracket. (*h to j*) Soon after the surgery and prior to the placement of any other orthodontic brackets, a palatal arch with a soldered spring was used to erupt the canine lingually and away from the root of the central incisor.

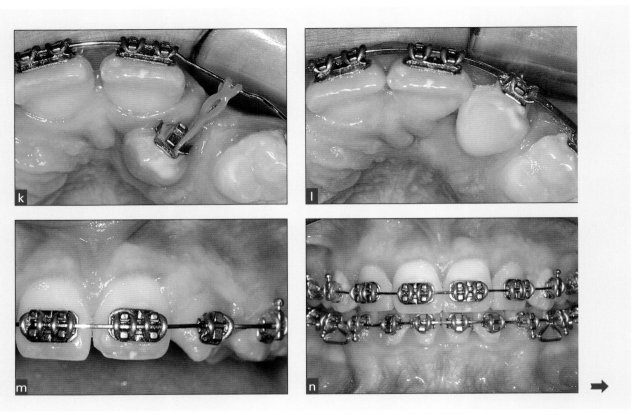

(**k to n**) Six months after surgery, brackets were placed on the remaining maxillary teeth, and the canine was moved into the dental arch. The maxillary right canine was also substituted for the right lateral incisor, and with the extraction of the two mandibular premolars, the occlusion could be finished in a Class I relationship.

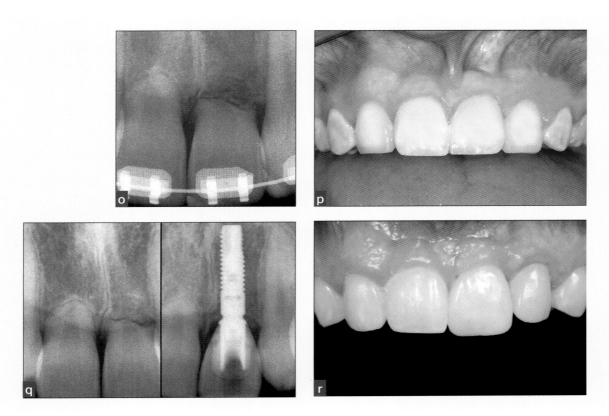

(o) A periapical radiograph taken toward the end of orthodontic treatment shows that no further resorption of the left central incisor had occurred after the canine was moved away from its root apex. (p) Composite restorations were placed on the incisal edges of the maxillary canines to simulate the appearance of lateral incisors. (q and r) Five years after orthodontic treatment, when the patient had completed her facial growth, the left central incisor was replaced with an implant and crown. (Restorative dentistry courtesy of Dr Gregg Kinzer, Seattle, Washington; implant courtesy of Dr Jim Janakievski, Tacoma, Washington.)

# References

1. Bass T. Observations on the misplaced upper canine tooth. Dent Pract 1967;18:25–33.

2. Johnston WD. Treatment of palatally impacted canine teeth. Am J Orthod 1969;56:589–596.

3. Lüdicke G, Harzer W, Tausche E. Incisor inclination—Risk factor for palatally-impacted canines. J Orofac Orthop 2008;69:357–364.

4. Al-Nimri KS, Bsoul E. Maxillary palatal canine impaction displacement in subjects with congenitally missing maxillary lateral incisors. Am J Orthod Dentofacial Orthop 2011;140:81–86.

5. Dachi S, Howell F. A survey of 3874 routine full mouth radiographs. Oral Surg Oral Med Oral Pathol 1961;14:1165–1169.

6. Ericson S, Kurol J. Radiographic assessment of maxillary canine eruption in children with clinical signs of eruption disturbances. Eur J Orthod 1986;8:133–140.

7. Liuk IW, Olive RJ, Griffin M, Monsour P. Maxillary lateral incisor morphology and palatally displaced canines: A case-controlled cone-beam volumetric tomography study. Am J Orthod Dentofacial Orthop 2013;143:522–526.

8. Motamedi MH, Tabatabaie FA, Nevi F, Shafeie HA, Fard BK, Hayati Z. Assessment of radiographic factors affecting surgical exposure and orthodontic alignment of impacted canines of the palate: A 15-year retrospective study. Oral Surg Oral Med Oral Pathol Oral Radiol Endod 2009;107:772–775.

9. Sajnani AK, King NM. Early prediction of maxillary canine impaction from panoramic radiographs. Am J Orthod Dentofacial Orthop 2012;142:45–51.

10. Schubert M, Baumert U. Alignment of impacted maxillary canines: Critical analysis of eruption path and treatment time. J Orofac Orthop 2009;70:200–212.

11. Ericson S, Kurol J. Early treatment of palatally erupting maxillary canines by extraction of the primary canines. Eur J Orthod 1988;10:283–295.

12. Jacobs SG. The impacted maxillary canine. Further observations on aetiology, radiographic localization, prevention/interception of impaction, and when to suspect impaction. Aust Dent J 1996;41:310–316.

13. Naoumova J, Kurol J, Kjellberg H. A systematic review of the interceptive treatment of palatally displaced maxillary canines. Eur J Orthod 2011;33:143–149.

14. Olive RJ. Orthodontic treatment of palatally impacted maxillary canines. Aust Orthod J 2002;18:64–70.

15. Baccetti T, Sigler LM, McNamara JA Jr. An RCT on treatment of palatally displaced canines with RME and/or a transpalatal arch. Eur J Orthod 2011;33:601–607.

16. Baccetti T, Mucedero M, Leonardi M, Cozza P. Interceptive treatment of palatal impaction of maxillary canines with rapid maxillary expansion: A randomized clinical trial. Am J Orthod Dentofacial Orthop 2009;136:657–661.

17. Yadav S, Upadhyay M, Uribe F, Nanda R. Palatally impacted maxillary canine with congenitally missing lateral incisors and midline diastema. Am J Orthod Dentofacial Orthop 2013;144:141–146.

18. Leonardi M, Armi P, Franchi, Baccetti T. Two interceptive approaches to palatally displaced canines: A prospective longitudinal study. Angle Orthod 2004;74:581–586.

19. Chapokas AR, Almas K, Schincaglia GP. The impacted maxillary canine: A proposed classification for surgical exposure. Oral Surg Oral Med Oral Pathol Oral Radiol Endod 2012;113:222–228.

20. Becker A, Zilberman Y. The palatally impacted canine: A new approach to treatment. Am J Orthod 1978;74:422–429.

21. Becker A, Kohavi D, Zilberman Y. Periodontal status following the alignment of palatally impacted canine teeth. Am J Orthod 1983;84:332–336.

22. Woloshyn H, Artun J, Kennedy DB, Joondeph DR. Pulpal and periodontal reactions to orthodontic alignment of palatally impacted canines. Angle Orthod 1994;64:257–264.

23. Hansson C, Rindler A. Periodontal conditions following surgical and orthodontic treatment of palatally impacted maxillary canines: A follow-up study. Angle Orthod 1998;68:167–172.

24. Ling K, Ho C, Kravchuk O, Olive R. Comparison of surgical and non-surgical methods of treating palatally impacted canines. II. Aesthetic outcomes. Aust Orthod J 2007;23:8–15.

25. Zasciurinskiene E, Bjerklin K, Smaliliene D, Sidlauskas A, Puisys A. Initial vertical and horizontal position of palatally impacted maxillary canine and effect on periodontal status following surgical-orthodontic treatment. Angle Orthod 2008;78:275–280.

26. Yadav S, Chen J, Upadhyay M, Jiang F, Roberts WE. Comparison of the force systems of 3 appliances on palatally impacted canines. Am J Orthod Dentofacial Orthop 2011;139:206–213.

27. Crescini A, Nieri M, Buti J, Baccetti T, Pini Prato GP. Orthodontic and periodontal outcomes of treated impacted maxillary canines. Angle Orthod 2007;77:571–577.

28. Clark D. The management of impacted canines: Free physiologic eruption. J Am Dent Assoc 1971;82:836–840.

29. Mathews DP, Kokich VG. Palatally impacted canines: The case for preorthodontic uncovering and autonomous eruption. Am J Orthod Dentofacial Orthop 2013;143:450–458.

30. Kokich VG. Preorthodontic uncovering and autonomous eruption of palatally impacted maxillary canines. Semin Orthod 2010;16:205–211.

31. Becker A, Chaushu G, Chaushu S. Analysis of failure in the treatment of impacted maxillary canines. Am J Orthod Dentofacial Orthop 2010;137:743–754.

32. Becker A, Chaushu S. Success rate and duration of orthodontic treatment for adult patients with palatally impacted maxillary canines. Am J Orthod Dentofacial Orthop 2003;124:509–514.

33. Ericson S, Kurol J. Resorption of maxillary lateral incisors caused by ectopic eruption of the canines. A clinical and radiographic analysis of predisposing factors. Am J Orthod Dentofacial Orthop 1988;94:503–513.

34. Ericson S, Kurol J. Incisor root resorptions due to ectopic maxillary canines imaged by computerized tomography: A comparative study in extracted teeth. Angle Orthod 2000;70:276–283.

35. Liu D, Zhang W, Zhang Z, Wu Y, Ma X. Localization of impacted maxillary canines and observation of adjacent incisor resorption with cone-beam computed tomography. Oral Surg Oral Med Oral Pathol Oral Radiol Endod 2008;105:91–98.

36. Owman-Moll P, Kurol J, Lundgren D. Repair of orthodontically induced root resorption in adolescents. Angle Orthod 1995;65:403–408.

37. Stewart J, Heo G, Glover K, Williamson P, Lam E, Major P. Factors that relate to treatment duration for patients with palatally impacted maxillary canines. Am J Orthod Dentofacial Orthop 2001;119:216–225.

38. Schmidt A, Kokich V. Periodontal response to early uncovering, autonomous eruption, and orthodontic alignment of palatally impacted maxillary canines. Am J Orthod Dentofacial Orthop 2007;131:449–455.

39. Ling KK, Ho CT, Kravchuk O, Olive RJ. Comparison of surgical and non-surgical methods of treating palatally impacted canines. I. Periodontal and pulpal outcomes. Aust Orthod J 2007;23:1–7.

40. Caprioglio A, Vanni A, Bolamperti L. Long-term periodontal response to orthodontic treatment of palatally impacted maxillary canines. Eur J Orthod 2013;35:323–328.

41. Smailiene D, Kavaliauskiene A, Pacauskiene I, Zasciurinskiene E, Bjerklin K. Palatally impacted maxillary canines: Choice of surgical-orthodontic treatment method does not influence post-treatment periodontal status. A controlled prospective study [epub ahead of print 24 Jan 2013]. Eur J Orthod.

42. Gharaibeh T, Al-Nimri K. Postoperative pain after surgical exposure of palatally impacted canines: Closed-eruption versus open-eruption, a prospective randomized study. Oral Surg Oral Med Oral Pathol Oral Radiol Endod 2008;106:339–342.

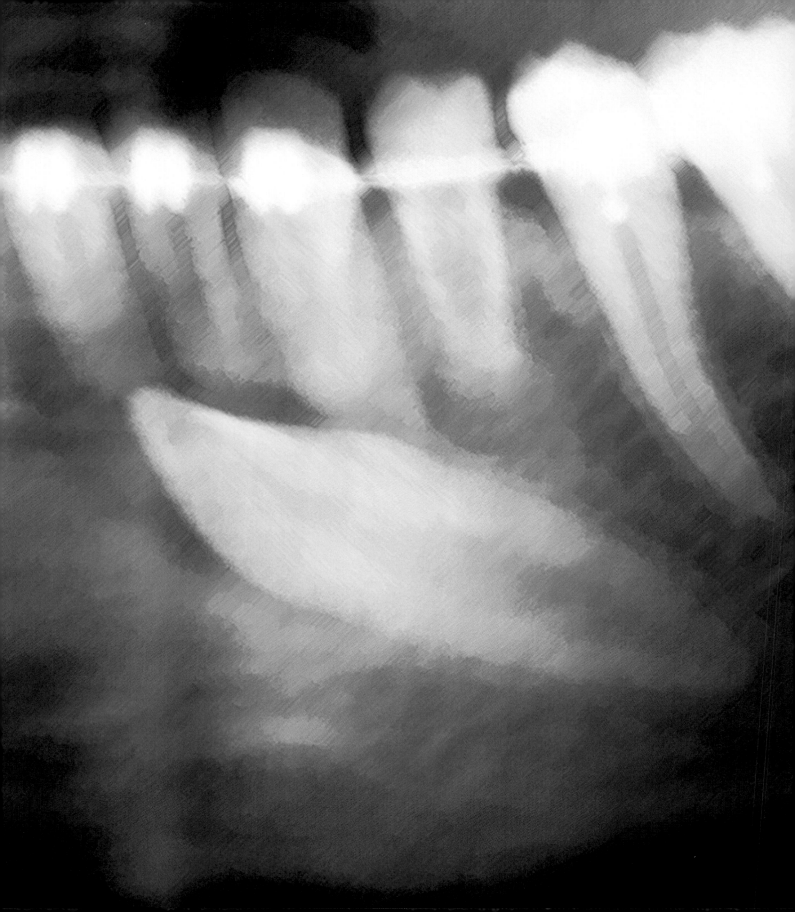

# Impacted Mandibular Canines

# 4

Mandibular canines are usually impacted in the midalveolar or labial position. Midalveolar impactions are usually vertically positioned in their normal location (see Fig 4-1). These can be uncovered easily with the closed eruption technique. When the canine is impacted labially, it is usually ectopically located and angled (see Figs 4-2 to 4-4). These will need to be left uncovered with an apically positioned flap. It is rare for the mandibular canine to be impacted lingually. Before any surgery is planned to uncover an impacted mandibular canine, it is imperative that the surgeon have adequate radiographs to make the proper diagnosis. It is important that the orthodontic appliances be in place and that the space be opened prior to surgery. The orthodontist should make the referral back to the surgeon when the patient is ready for the uncovering. The primary tooth and any supernumerary teeth should be extracted at the time of the uncovering.

Fig 4-1 ) Impacted mandibular right canine caused by a supernumerary tooth.

**Fig 4-1** ) **Impacted mandibular right canine caused by a supernumerary tooth.**

(a) This adolescent girl had a supernumerary tooth positioned adjacent to her mandibular right canine that had caused the impaction of this tooth. (b) The mandibular right primary canine and supernumerary tooth were removed, orthodontic brackets were placed, and the space was opened in the mandibular right canine region, but the permanent canine did not erupt. (c) A closed eruption technique was used. A midcrestal incision was made and a pedicle flap reflected. Bone was removed to expose the crown of the canine. (d) A chain was bonded to the incisal edge of the canine, and the flap was repositioned, allowing the chain to exit through the midcrestal incision.

## Vertically Impacted Canines

To uncover the midalveolar and labially impacted mandibular canine, the closed eruption technique can be employed if the tooth is fairly vertical and not ectopically positioned (Fig 4-1). A crestal incision is made with conservative reflection to gain access to the impacted tooth. Sometimes vertical incisions are needed to gain adequate access for appropriate bone removal. The tooth is uncovered and enough bone removed to expose the crown of the tooth. The area is isolated with hemostatic agents so there is a clean, dry field. The tooth is etched and a bonding agent placed so that a chain can be bonded to it. It is easiest to bond the chain directly to the tooth without using a bracket (see Fig 4-1d). The flap is repositioned and sutured. The chain will exit through the midcrestal incision and is attached to a bracket on an adjacent tooth. The orthodontist can initiate tooth movement 2 weeks later.

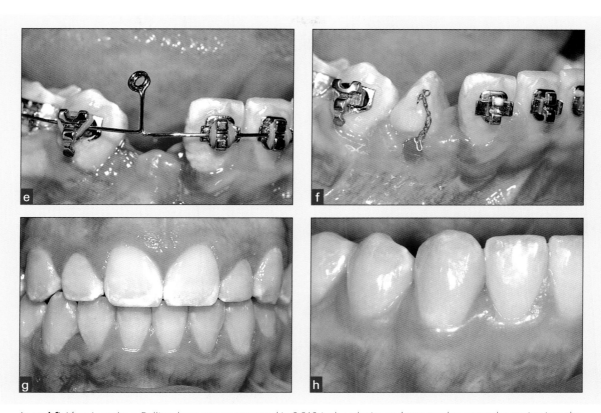

(*e and f*) After 6 weeks, a Ballista loop was constructed in 0.018-inch archwire and was used to erupt the canine into the center of the alveolar ridge. (*g*) The canine was bracketed and rotated into position, and the orthodontic treatment was completed. (*h*) A 5-year posttreatment photograph shows how natural the gingiva and mucosa appear when a tooth is erupted using the closed eruption technique.

A Ballista spring (see Fig 4-1e) is the best device to erupt this type of impacted canine. Once the tooth has been erupted, it can be bracketed so that final movement and finishing can be accomplished. This type of orthodontic force will mimic the natural eruption pathway. It will erupt the tooth through the center of the edentulous ridge, which will result in a normal gingival complex without any recession (see Fig 4-1h).

**Fig 4-2** ) **Labially impacted and ectopically positioned mandibular right canine.**

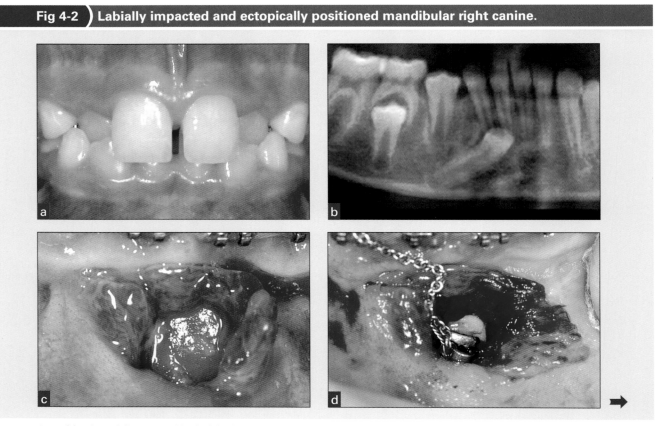

*(a and b)* This adolescent girl had a labially impacted mandibular right canine that was ectopically positioned mesial to the mandibular right lateral incisor. *(c)* A flap was reflected to expose the labial bone, which was covering the impacted canine. *(d)* The bone was removed, exposing the canine crown, and a cleat was bonded to the tooth, with an auxiliary chain extending into the oral cavity.

Labially impacted canines are often positioned ectopically and angled (Fig 4-2). These teeth must be left uncovered with an apically positioned flap.

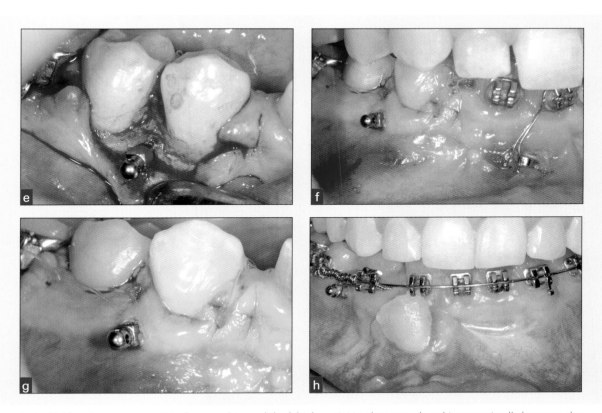

**(e to h)** After the canine was initially moved toward the labial, a mini-implant was placed interproximally between the first and second premolars to be used as anchorage to retract the canine. (Orthodontics courtesy of Dr Doug Knight, Tacoma, Washington.)

# Horizontally Impacted Canines

Very infrequently, the canine will be impacted on the labial in a horizontal position. If it is not displaced such that the tip of the tooth is at or past the midline, it can be uncovered, orthodontically forced to erupt, and moved into its proper position. However, if the impacted canine is too close to or past the midline (Fig 4-3), it may be difficult or impossible for the orthodontist to move it. Sometimes extraction may be the treatment of choice when all factors are considered. The risk of damage to the adjacent teeth needs to be evaluated if tooth movement is contemplated.

The orthodontist must first open space for the horizontally impacted canine. Once the appropriate space has been created, the patient can be referred to the surgeon to uncover the impacted tooth.

If there is inadequate attached gingiva, the area should be grafted before uncovering the impacted tooth (see Fig 4-3c). Horizontally impacted mandibular canines that are not too close to the midline can be uncovered with an apically positioned flap. It is imperative that these impactions be left uncovered so that the orthodontist can apply appropriate mechanics to erupt them (see Fig 4-3). The orthodontist should first erupt the tooth labially (see Figs 4-3c to 4-3e). The tooth can then be rebracketed and moved into ideal position.

Extra orthodontic anchorage (ie, temporary anchorage devices [TADs]) can be used to facilitate movement of these very difficult impactions. The TAD can be placed between the premolars to facilitate the movement. The TAD can be placed in gingiva, near the mucogingival junction, by a punch technique or reflection of a miniflap for better visualization of the bone for more accurate drilling and placement (see Fig 4-2).

Placement of a bracket and a dressing is usually required to keep these teeth uncovered due to their apical depth in the vestibule. Orthodontics can be initiated 4 to 6 weeks later.

## Fig 4-3    Ectopically positioned and horizontally impacted mandibular canines.

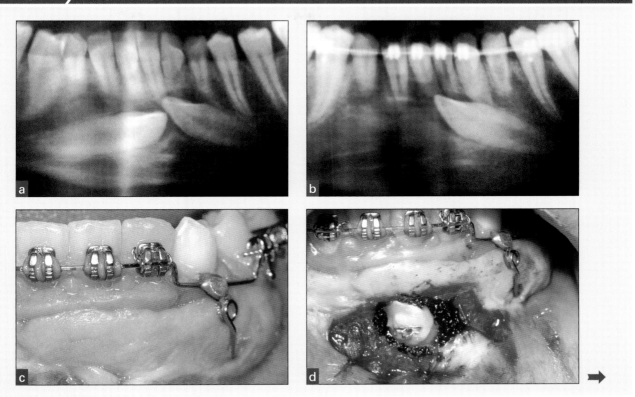

**(a)** This 13-year-old boy had two ectopically positioned and impacted mandibular canines. **(b)** Because of its hopeless position, the mandibular right canine was extracted, and the right primary canine was allowed to remain to maintain the alveolar ridge for a possible future implant. **(c)** An autogenous gingival graft was placed to augment the labial gingiva. **(d)** Eight weeks later, a pedicle flap was elevated and bone was removed to expose the mandibular left canine. A bracket was bonded to the canine, and the flap was apically positioned, leaving the canine crown exposed.

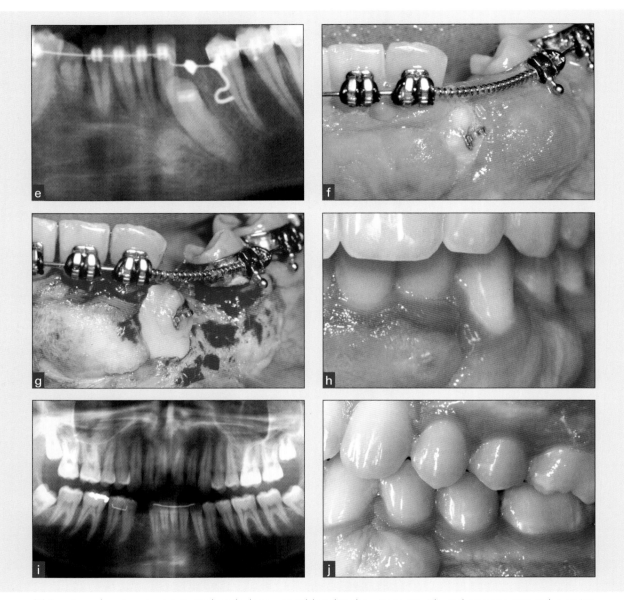

**(e)** A rectangular wire was constructed, and a loop was soldered to the wire to provide anchorage to retract the canine distally. After the canine had been partially retracted **(f)**, a gingivoplasty was performed to aid in final tooth movement **(g and h)**. **(i and j)** Five-year posttreatment radiograph and occlusion. (Orthodontics courtesy of Dr Tim Quinn, Gig Harbor, Washington.)

**Fig 4-4** ) **Labially and mesially impacted mandibular left canine exposed via split-thickness flap.**

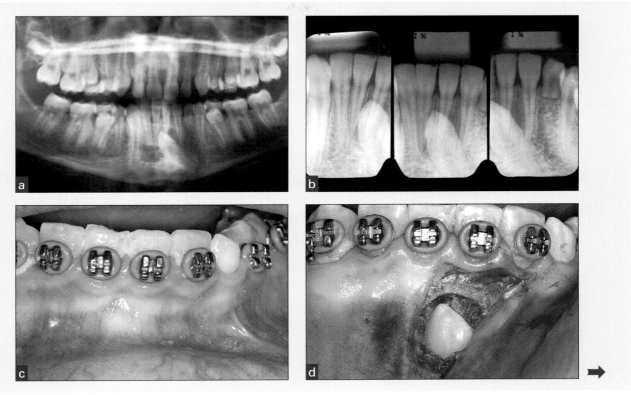

(a) This adolescent boy had a labially and mesially impacted mandibular left canine. The periapical radiographs (b) and intraoral palpation (c) confirmed that the canine was positioned labially. (d) A split-thickness pedicle flap was reflected, and bone was removed from the crown of the impacted tooth.

# Tissue Grafting

These teeth should be reevaluated during and after orthodontic movement. Occasionally, they will require gingival augmentation with a free gingival graft or connective tissue grafting. This may occur when the impacted tooth is ectopically and apically positioned at or below the mucogingival junction. In the patient shown in Fig 4-3, there was inadequate gingiva prior to uncovering, and a gingival graft was placed prior to uncovering. A minor gingivectomy was required midway through the eruption process to aid the orthodontist in final positioning. In the patient shown in Fig 4-4, however, no grafting was accomplished, and moderate recession occurred during the eruption process. This type of recession is easily treated with a connective tissue graft.

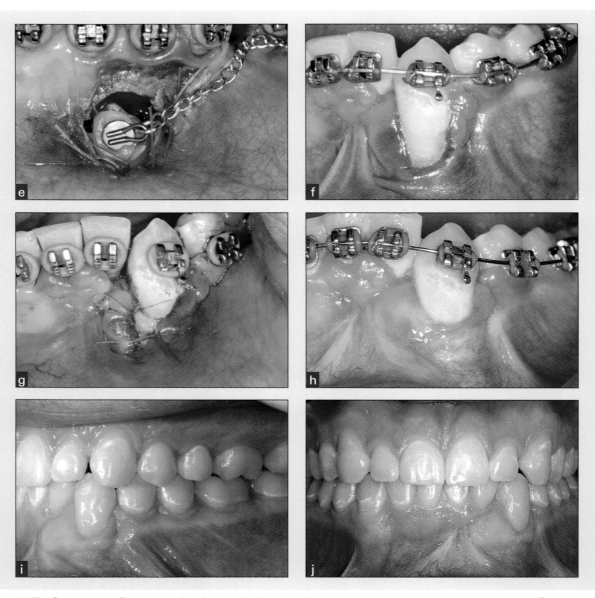

(e) The flap was apically positioned and sutured with resorbable sutures. A bracket was bonded to the labial of the canine, and the end of the chain was temporarily secured to the mandibular premolar bracket. The canine was retracted orthodontically using a mandibular lingual arch for anchorage. (f) Eventually the canine was bracketed, and archwires were used to erupt the crown occlusally. Moderate recession had occurred during the eruptive movement (f), so a connective tissue graft was placed (g) and allowed to heal for 3 months (h) prior to further orthodontic movement. (i and j) Seven years after bracket removal, the canine position and soft tissue attachment have remained stable. (Orthodontics courtesy of Dr Doug Knight, Tacoma, Washington.)

# Recommended Reading

Agarwal S, Yadav S, Shah NV, Valiathan A, Uribe F, Nanda R. Correction of bilateral impacted mandibular canines with a lip bumper for anchorage reinforcement. Am J Orthod Dentofacial Orthop 2013;143:393–403.

Almeida RC, Carvalho FA, Almeida MA, Capelli J Jr. Orthodontic management of a patient with impacted and transposed mandibular canines. World J Orthod 2009;10:345–349.

Aras MH, Halicioğlu K, Yavuz MS, Çağlaroğlu M. Evaluation of surgical-orthodontic treatments on impacted mandibular canines. Med Oral Patol Oral Cir Bucal 2011;16:e925–e928.

Auluck A, Nagpal A, Setty S, Pai KM, Sunny J. Transmigration of impacted mandibular canines—Report of 4 cases. J Can Dent Assoc 2006;72:249–252.

Bahl R, Singla J, Gupta M, Malhotra A. Aberrantly placed impacted mandibular canine. Contemp Clin Dent 2013;4:217–219.

Buyukkurt MC, Aras MH, Çağlaroğlu M. Extraoral removal of a transmigrant mandibular canine associated with a dentigerous cyst. Quintessence Int 2008;39:767–770.

Buyukkurt MC, Aras MH, Çağlaroğlu M, Gungormus M. Transmigrant mandibular canines. J Oral Maxillofac Surg 2007;65:2025–2029.

Cabrera Diaz JR. Impacted mandibular canines. Int J Orthod Milwaukee 2011;22(3):25–30.

Camilleri S, Scerri E. Transmigration of mandibular canines—A review of the literature and a report of five cases. Angle Orthod 2003;73:753–762.

Cowman SC, Wootton WR. Bilateral impaction of mandibular canines. N Z Dent J 1979;75:113–114.

Crescini A, Baccetti T, Rotundo R, Mancini EA, Prato GP. Tunnel technique for the treatment of impacted mandibular canines. Int J Periodontics Restorative Dent 2009;29:213–218.

Edstrom EJ, Smith MM, Taney K. Extraction of the impacted mandibular canine tooth in the dog. J Vet Dent 2013;30:56–61.

González-Sánchez MA, Berini-Aytés L, Gay-Escoda C. Transmigrant impacted mandibular canines: A retrospective study of 15 cases. J Am Dent Assoc 2007;138:1450–1455.

Gunashekhar M, Rohini M. Transmigration of mandibular canines: A rare case report and review of the literature. J Dent Child (Chic) 2011;78:19–23.

Holla A, Saify M, Parashar S. Transmigration of impacted mandibular canines and its assocation with malocclusion and morphology: An analysis of seven cases. Orthodontics (Chic) 2012;13:156–165.

Hudson AP, Harris AM, Mohamed N. Early identification and management of mandibular canine ectopia. SADJ 2011;66:462–464.

Joshi MR. Transmigrant mandibular canines: A record of 28 cases and a retrospective review of the literature. Angle Orthod 2001;72:12–22.

Kokich VG, Mathews DP. Surgical and orthodontic management of impacted teeth. Dent Clin North Am 1993;37:181–204.

Kontham U, Kontham R, Mistry J. Transmigration of mandibular canines in siblings: A case report. Quintessence Int 2012;43:45–49.

Mupparapu M. Patterns of intra-osseous transmigration and ectopic eruption of mandibular canines: Review of literature and report of nine additional cases. Dentomaxillofac Radiol 2002;31:355–360.

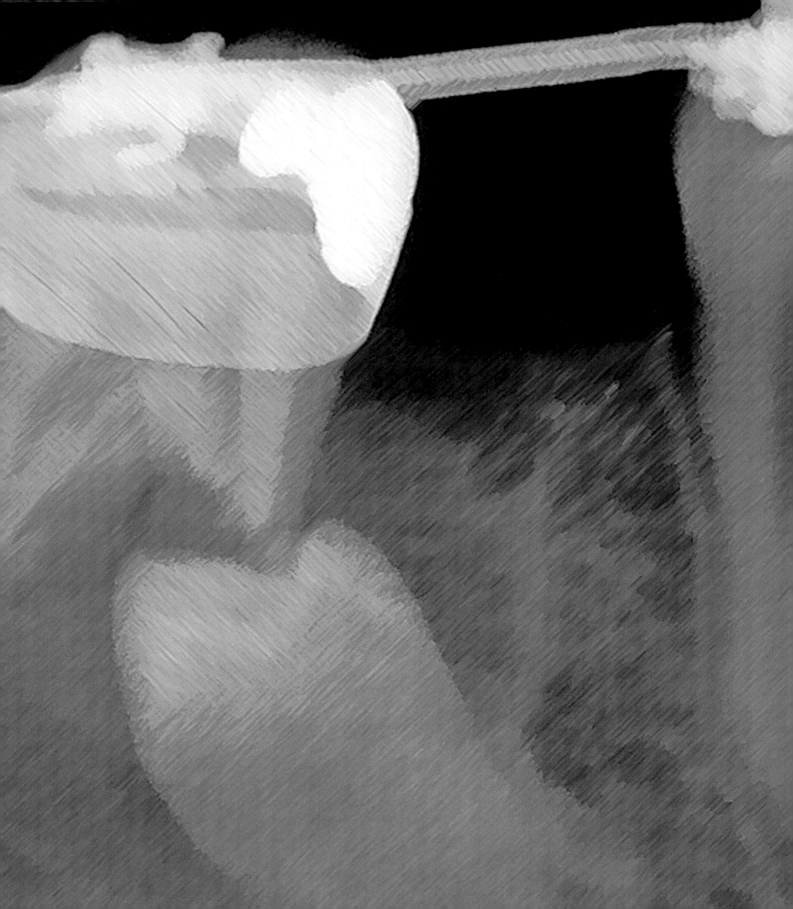

# Impacted Premolars

The most commonly impacted premolar is the mandibular second premolar (Figs 5-1 and 5-2). Impaction of maxillary premolars is uncommon. Both maxillary and mandibular premolar impactions are typically located in a midalveolar or lingual/palatal position. An impacted mandibular premolar usually can be palpated if it is positioned lingually (see Fig 5-3d). Appropriate radiographs should be taken to ascertain the exact location of the tooth (see Figs 5-2c and 5-2d). If the tooth cannot be palpated, it is usually in a mid-alveolar or palatal position. It is uncommon to find an impacted maxillary or mandibular premolar on the buccal surface. Impacted premolars can be uncovered with one of two techniques: the closed eruption technique or the preorthodontic uncovering technique.

### Fig 5-1  Horizontally impacted mandibular right second premolar.

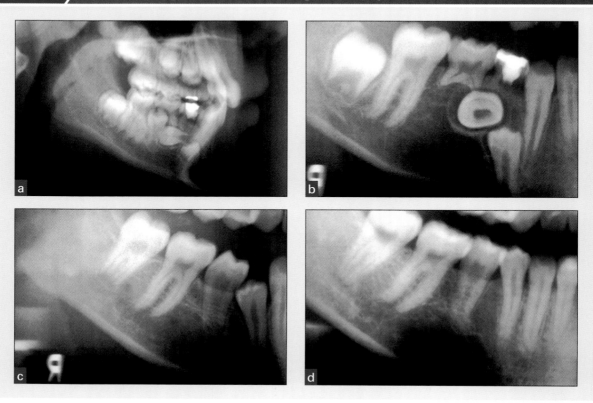

(a and b) This patient was 10 years, 7 months old and in the mixed dentition. Her mandibular right second premolar was impacted horizontally, with the crown directed distally. The impacted second premolar was inhibiting the eruption of the mandibular right first premolar. The treatment involved extraction of both first and second primary molars and the placement of a mandibular lingual arch to maintain the position of the first molar. (c) By the time the patient was 13 years old, the mandibular right second premolar had erupted autonomously into the dental arch, which had allowed the first premolar to also erupt into its normal position. Orthodontic treatment was initiated to correct the rotation of the second premolar and complete the eruption of the first premolar. (d) After orthodontic treatment, when the patient was 14 years, 10 months old, the roots and crowns of the previously impacted teeth were in their proper position.

## Fig 5-2 ) Impacted mandibular left second premolar.

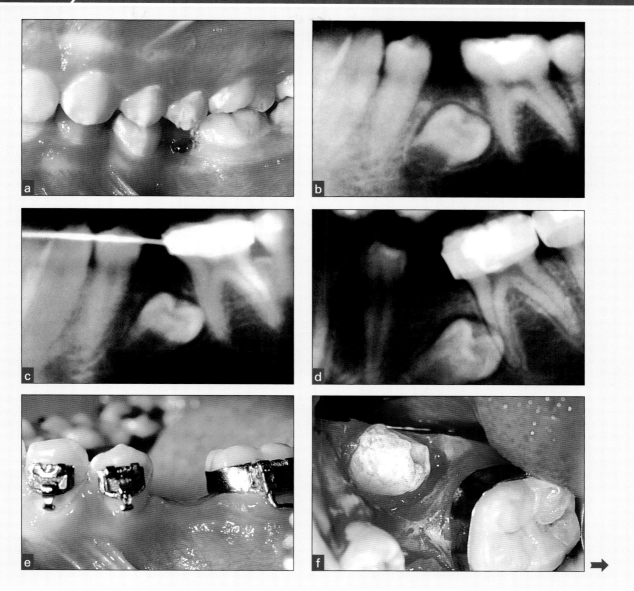

(a) All of this 13-year-old girl's teeth had erupted except for the mandibular left second premolar. (b) The radiograph at age 13 years showed that the second premolar crown had developed but that the root had just begun to form. It was decided that uncovering the tooth at this time could arrest further root development. (c) A lingual arch was placed to maintain the molar position, and the patient was observed for 2 years. (d) When the patient was 15 years old, the root of the mandibular second premolar had developed, and orthodontic treatment was initiated. (e) Initially, space was opened orthodontically for the second premolar crown. (f) A lingual flap was reflected, and bone was removed from over the crown of the tooth.

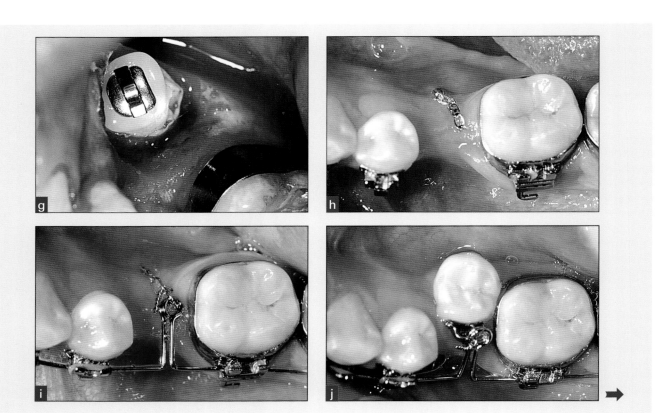

**(g)** The tooth was in a rotated position with the lingual surface facing occlusally, so a bracket was bonded to the lingual surface of the tooth. **(h)** A gold chain was attached to the bracket. A fenestration was made through the gingival portion of the flap. The flap was repositioned, and the chain exited through the tissue fenestration. **(i)** A Ballista spring was constructed using 0.018-inch round archwire. The spring was activated by attaching it to the gold chain near the crest of the alveolar ridge. **(j)** As the spring moved coronally, it forced the crown of the premolar to erupt.

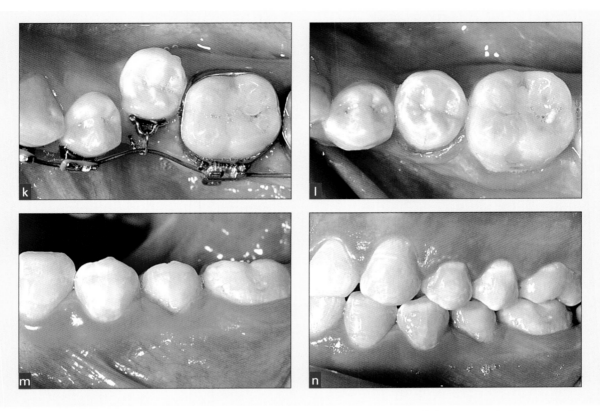

*(k)* Once the crown had erupted through the gingiva, it was advantageous to use a nickel-titanium archwire to move the crown buccally and into position. *(l to n)* No attempt was made to rotate the crown of the premolar. After removal of the appliance, a composite resin restoration was bonded to the buccal surface of the premolar to create an occlusal cusp to make contact with the opposing maxillary second premolar.

## Closed Eruption Technique

When a mandibular premolar is impacted lingually, a full-thickness lingual flap is reflected from the canine to the mesial of the second molar (Fig 5-3). Occasionally, a vertical incision will be needed when the impacted tooth is positioned near the apices of the adjacent teeth. Careful bone removal is accomplished to create an access wider than the dimension of the impacted crown so that it can be extricated from its bony crypt. This must be performed carefully, because the tooth may be impacted near the mesial root of the first molar (see Fig 5-5d).

Once the tooth has been isolated, a gold chain is bonded to the coronal aspect (Figs 5-4 and 5-5). The flaps are repositioned and sutured. The chain will exit through the incision at the midcrestal region and should be attached to an adjacent bracket (see Figs 5-4 and 5-5). An eruptive orthodontic force can be applied 1 to 2 weeks later. If the premolar is in the midalveolar position, it will erupt quickly with application of a Ballista spring.

**Fig 5-3** ) **Ectopic, lingually impacted mandibular second premolar.**

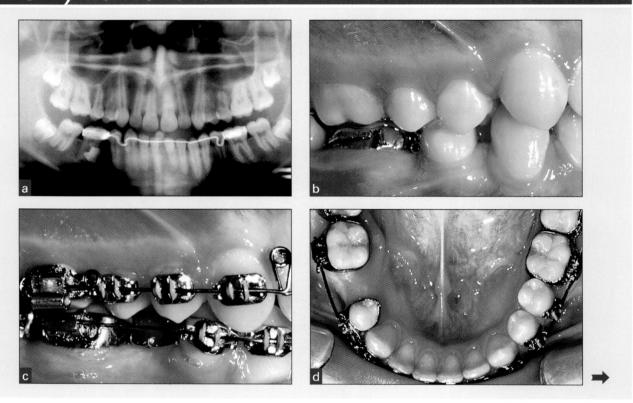

*(a and b)* This adolescent boy was 14 years, 2 months old. The mandibular right second premolar was delayed in its development, so a lingual arch was placed at an earlier age to maintain the first molar position until root development of the second premolar was complete. *(c and d)* Orthodontic appliances were placed on all teeth, and initially space was opened between the mandibular right first premolar and first molar. At that time, the patient was referred to have the lingually impacted second premolar uncovered.

Infrequently, the impacted premolar will be locked under the root of the first molar. In this case, special orthodontic mechanics will be needed to erupt it (see Fig 5-5). In such cases when the tooth is badly impacted near the apex of the first molar, some root resorption may occur as the tooth is moved. The orthodontic force and direction are critical in extricating the tooth from beneath the crown of the first molar without causing damage to its already resorbed mesial root. This resorption will cease after the tooth is erupted because the premolar will no longer be putting pressure on the mesial root of the molar (see Fig 5-5).

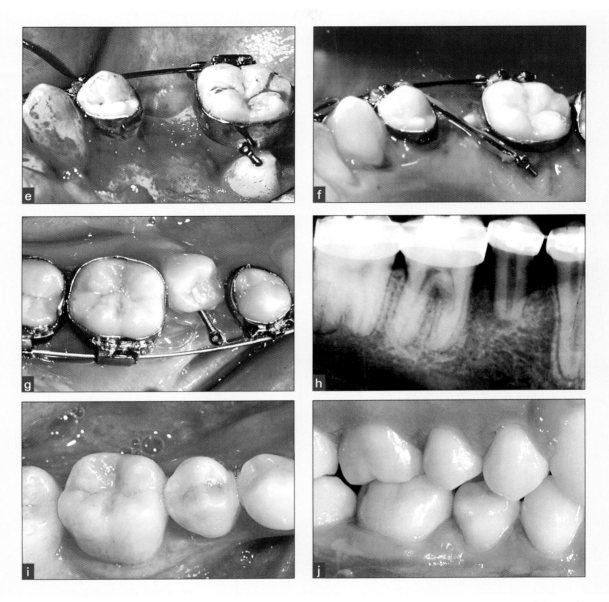

**(e)** A lingual flap was reflected from the canine to the second molar. Bone was removed from over the crown of the tooth. In this particular case, a pin was attached to the buccal surface of the tooth to create a secure attachment to the tooth. The flap was repositioned so that the pin exited through the marginal gingiva. **(f and g)** Three weeks after surgery, an elastomeric chain was attached from the pin to the archwire to move the crown mesially. After the crown had cleared the lingual surface of the first molar, the pin was removed, a band was placed on the second premolar, and the crown was moved buccally. **(h)** After the root was aligned, the root length was shorter than normal. **(i and j)** One year after ortho-dontics, the position of the second premolar has remained stable.

## Fig 5-4  Use of a gold chain to erupt an impacted premolar.

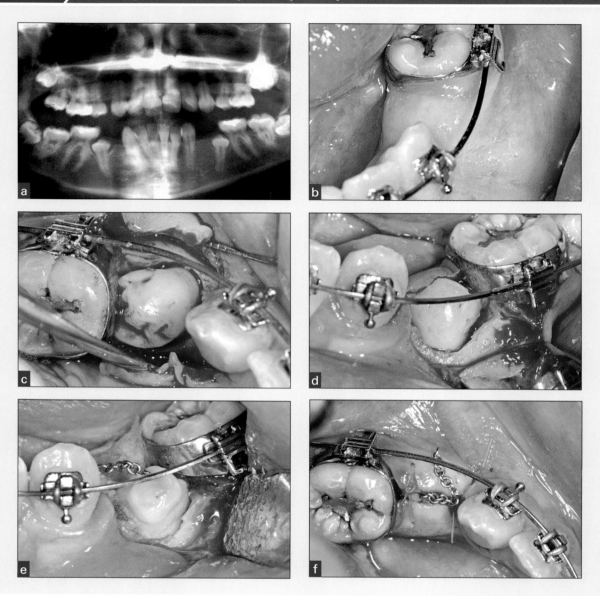

(*a and b*) Despite the prior extraction of all first premolars to address severe arch length deficiencies, the mandibular second premolars were impacted against the mesial surfaces of the first molars. Space was prepared for the impacted teeth, and the arch was stabilized with an edgewise wire in anticipation of the surgical procedures. (*c and d*) A midcrestal incision was made in the edentulous area, and full-thickness flaps were reflected. Bone was removed to expose the clinical crown of the mandibular second premolar. (*e*) The enamel was etched, a bonding agent was placed, and a gold chain was bonded directly to the buccal cusp of the premolar. (*f*) The flaps were repositioned and sutured with resorbable sutures. The chain exited through the midcrestal incision line. A Ballista spring could be used to erupt the premolar through the crest of the ridge.

## Fig 5-5 ) Impacted premolar causing root resorption of the first molar.

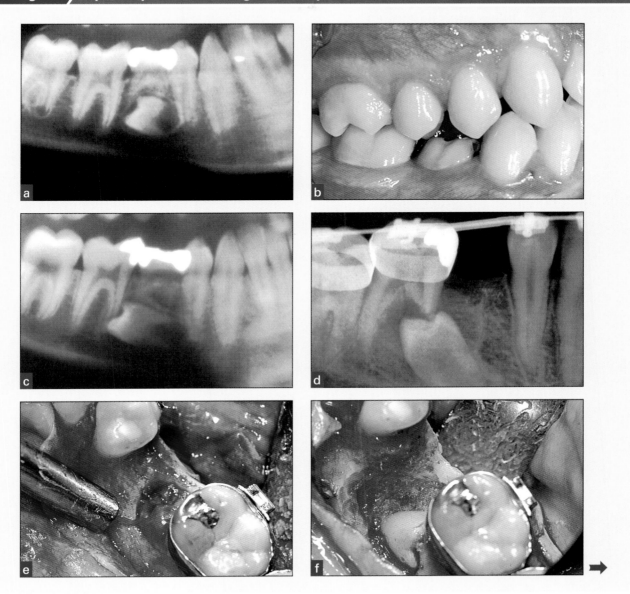

(a) This adolescent boy was 12½ years old. The development of his mandibular right second premolar was delayed, and the crown was directed distally. It was decided to wait for further root development before beginning orthodontics. (b and c) When the patient was 15 years old, the root had begun development, so orthodontic treatment was initiated, and the primary molar was extracted. (d) Six months after initiating orthodontic treatment, it was time to uncover the second premolar. By this time, the premolar crown had turned, begun to erupt, and was causing significant resorption of the mesial root of the first molar. (e and f) A lingual flap was reflected, and bone was removed carefully to uncover the crown of the premolar.

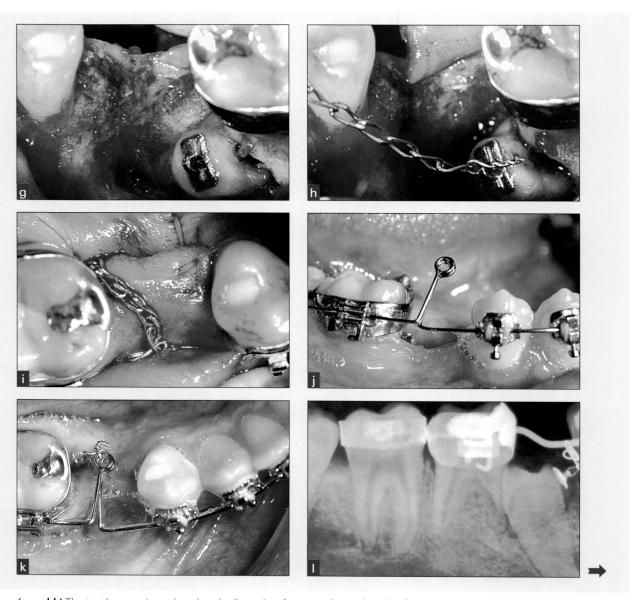

(*g and h*) The tooth was oriented so that the lingual surface was directed occlusally. A cleat was bonded to the lingual surface, and a gold chain was ligated to the cleat. (*i*) The flap was repositioned, and the gold chain exited through a fenestration that had been made in the lingual portion of the flap. (*j to l*) A Ballista loop was created in an 0.018-inch archwire. The loop was constructed to deliver a mesially and occlusally directed force to move the second premolar crown away from the resorbing root of the first molar.

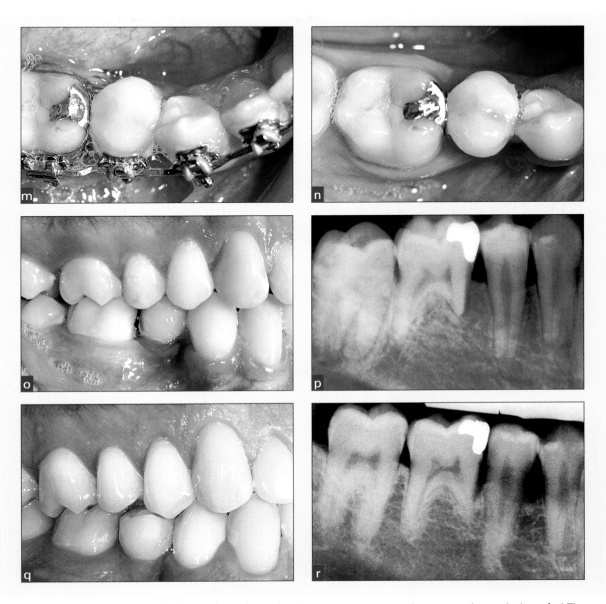

(m) After the premolar crown had moved into the oral cavity, no attempt was made to rotate the tooth. (n and o) The appliances were removed, and the buccal surface was restored with composite resin to create a cusp to contact the maxillary premolar in occlusion. (p) A radiograph taken after orthodontic treatment shows that the mesial root of the first molar did not resorb any further after the second premolar had been moved. (q and r) Twenty-two years later, the occlusion and the root length of the second premolar and first molar have remained stable.

# Preorthodontic Uncovering Technique

When a maxillary premolar is impacted in the palate or in the midalveolar area, the preorthodontic uncovering technique can be used (Fig 5-6). A flap is reflected from the mesial of the first molar to the canine. Appropriate bone removal is accomplished to completely expose the crown of the tooth, and an orthodontic bracket is bonded to the coronal or occlusal aspect of the premolar (see Fig 5-6f). The flap is repositioned, and, prior to suturing, it is scalloped to expose enough of the crown so that a dressing can be applied to the bracket (see Fig 5-6g). The dressing can be removed a few weeks later, unless the premolar is impacted very high in the palate, in which case the dressing is left until the tooth erupts enough on its own. When the premolar is near the surface of the palate, there is less concern that the tissue will re-cover the tooth, so the dressing can be removed. Occasionally, the dressing will need to remain for 2 to 3 months. When the tooth has erupted significantly through the palatal tissue, the orthodontist can begin active movement.

# Orthodontic Mechanics to Erupt an Impacted Premolar

The choice of orthodontic mechanics necessary to erupt a premolar will depend on the orientation of the root and the vertical depth of the impacted crown. If the impacted premolar is located in a midalveolar position and oriented nearly vertical in the alveolus, the authors recommend use of a Ballista spring to erupt the tooth vertically and within the labial and lingual plates of the alveolar bone (see Fig 5-2i). The length of the Ballista spring should be equal to the distance from the labial archwire to the center of the alveolar ridge. In this way, the tooth will erupt vertically and more efficiently. Once the tooth has erupted through the gingiva at the crest of the ridge, a bracket can be placed on the tooth so that the crown can be positioned properly relative to the adjacent teeth.

If the premolar crown is positioned on the palatal or lingual surface and lies lingual to the first molar roots, then the force of a Ballista spring is difficult to orient properly to facilitate tooth movement. In these situations, an elastomeric chain is helpful to encourage movement of the tooth toward the center of the alveolus and mesial to the first molar (see Fig 5-3f). It is important to make certain that there is sufficient anchorage to support the elastomeric chain. In some situations, it is advantageous to place a lingual or palatal arch from which to anchor the elastomeric chain. In other cases, a miniscrew can be used to help anchor the force of the elastomeric chain. In either case, it is important that the clinician does not direct the force in a way that causes damage to the first molar roots.

Occasionally, the eruptive path of the impacted mandibular second premolar crown will become diverted distally and cause resorption of the first molar roots (see Figs 5-5c and 5-5d). Although this is not typical, once this has occurred, it is important to move the impacted crown away from the first molar as soon as possible to avoid irreparable damage and potential loss of the first molar. In these cases, a Ballista spring is typically not useful. The preferred mechanism for moving the premolar crown away from the first molar roots is an elastomeric chain or a nickel-titanium spring attached to a lingual arch, a palatal arch, or a miniscrew.

## Fig 5-6 ) Impacted premolars in a patient with Down syndrome.

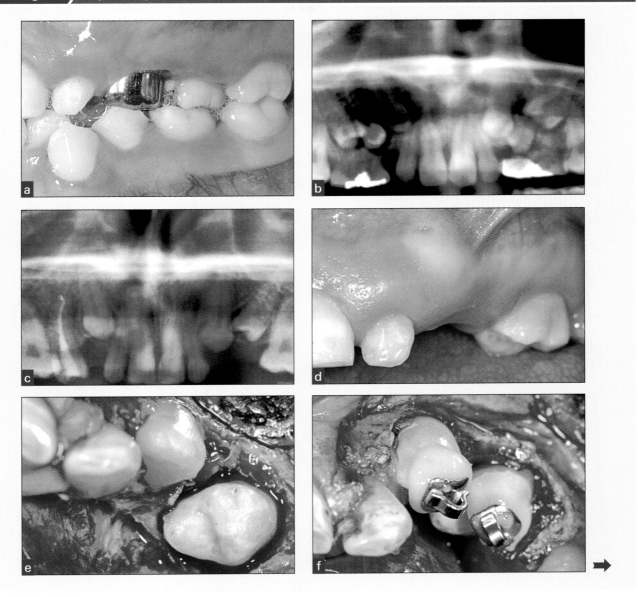

(a and b) This adolescent girl was 14 years, 8 months old and had a mild form of Down syndrome. Despite complete root formation, the eruption of her maxillary right and left premolars and canines was delayed significantly. In addition, she had a pronounced maxillary arch length deficiency. The four maxillary primary molars and the right and left first premolars were extracted at that time. (c and d) Six years later, when the patient was 20 years, 7 months old, the maxillary left second premolar and canine had shown little eruptive progress. At that time, the patient was referred for uncovering of the impacted teeth. (e and f) The maxillary right canine and second premolar were midalveolar impactions. Buccal and palatal flaps were reflected, and bone was removed from the crowns of the teeth. Cleats were bonded on the incisal edge of the canine and buccal cusp tip of the second premolar, and the flaps were repositioned.

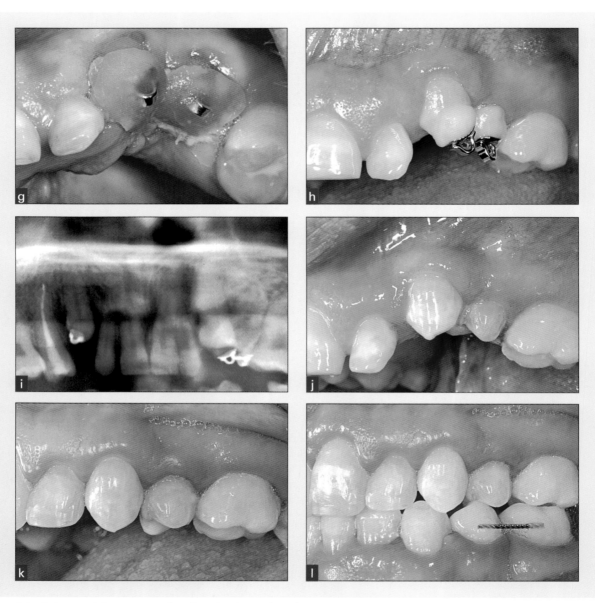

(g) A light-cured dressing was placed on the cleats. (h and i) One year later, the canine and second premolar showed considerable eruption compared with the previous 6 years. (j to l) The cleats were removed, orthodontic brackets were bonded to all teeth, and the canine and second premolar were erupted into occlusion.

As stated earlier, if the impacted second premolar is not in a midalveolar position, it is typically positioned either toward the lingual or palatal of the roots of the first molar. The patient in Fig 5-3 is an example of this type of situation. In such cases, the authors do not recommend a Ballista spring to erupt the tooth toward the center of the alveolar ridge. A directive force of a Ballista spring is difficult to control in this situation. Therefore, in this case, the author (VGK) chose to use an elastomeric chain to move the crown of the second premolar first toward the mesial and then into the dental arch. In some of these cases, it is difficult to direct the premolar away from the roots of the molar to avoid root damage. In fact, it is almost inevitable that some root resorption will occur on the lingual surfaces of the mandibular molar roots during this type of tooth movement. However, researchers have shown that once the crown of the impacted tooth has been moved away from the root, cementoblasts will differentiate from mesenchymal cells and deposit cellular cementum on the surface of the root to repair the resorptive areas.

Occasionally, when a mandibular or maxillary second premolar is impacted toward the lingual surface, the surface that the surgeon first sees when the bone is removed from the premolar crown is the lingual surface (see Figs 5-5g and 5-5h). Therefore, the surgeon often must bond a gold chain or attachment to the lingual surface. As the tooth is pulled toward the mesial in these situations, the authors recommend rotating the tooth; once the tooth enters the center of the alveolar ridge, the crown is often rotated 180 degrees. This situation occurred in Fig 5-2 and 5-5. In both cases, the author (VGK) chose to leave the crown rotated 180 degrees, with the lingual surface positioned buccally. Although the tooth could have been rotated orthodontically, the risk of relapse of the rotation would have been high due to the attachment of the circumferential transseptal gingival fiber network. In the patients in Figs 5-2 and 5-5, the author bonded a composite resin buccal cusp on the rotated premolar crown so that it would appear more natural and have better occlusal contact with the opposing dental arch (see Fig 5-5n).

The patient illustrated in Fig 5-5 not only had a difficult mandibular second premolar impaction but also significant resorption of the first molar root (see Fig 5-5d), which was discovered when orthodontic treatment was initiated and the author (VGK) was preparing to have the premolar crown uncovered. At the time of uncovering of the tooth, the author was concerned that either the first molar pulp would become nonvital during the surgery or that the significance of the root resorption could produce a severe periodontal osseous defect during eruption of the second premolar. Therefore, the prognosis for the first molar was guarded due to these possibilities. However, even if the first molar were lost, it would still be beneficial to at least erupt the second premolar to encourage vertical development of the bony ridge in that area, in case an implant would be needed later to replace the first molar. However, to the author's surprise, after the second premolar was extricated from beneath the mesial roots of the first molar, the root resorption stopped, the bone filled into the furcation of the first molar, and both the first molar and second premolar maintained their pulpal vitality (see Figs 5-5o and 5-5p). As stated earlier, once the pressure against the root is removed, the cementoblasts deposit cellular or reparative cementum over the resorbed surfaces of the root.

# Autonomous Eruption

In some situations, a badly impacted second premolar will erupt autonomously if one or two primary molars in the area are extracted. In the patient in Fig 5-7, the primary molar was ankylosed, and it impeded the second premolar from erupting. The premolar became horizontally impacted. Extraction of the ankylosed primary molar allowed for autonomous eruption of the impacted second premolar.

There are few reports in the literature regarding this possibility, and most references to autonomous eruption are from single case reports or small case series. The possibility for self-correction is not predictable, but it is certainly worth trying, especially if the impaction is horizontal and the patient is still in the mixed dentition. In the patients illustrated in Figs 5-1 and 5-6, a mandibular and maxillary second premolar, respectively, was horizontally impacted. In both cases, the only treatment was to extract the primary second molars, place a lingual or palatal arch, and observe the results. In each case, the second premolar erupted autonomously. In fact, these teeth erupted until they were nearly in ideal position relative to the adjacent teeth. Autonomous eruption is certainly not predictable, but it is definitely worth attempting in the patient who is in the mixed dentition and has several years until all permanent teeth will erupt.

**Fig 5-7** Impacted maxillary right second premolar due to ankylosis of the primary second molar.

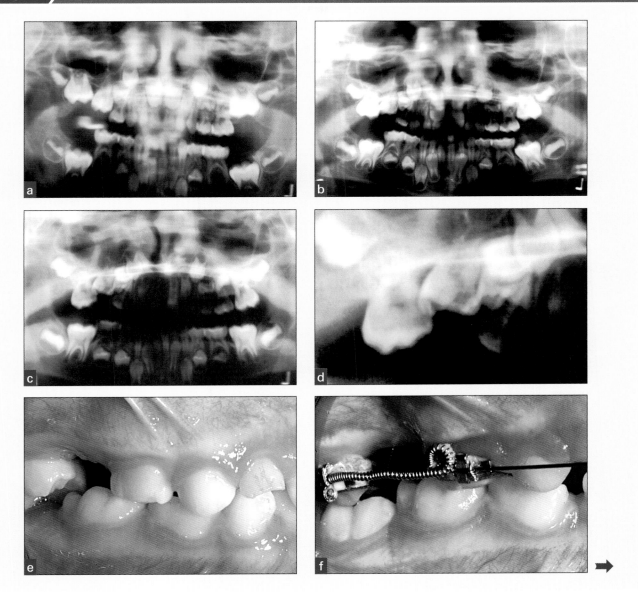

**(a)** This 5½-year-old girl's maxillary right primary second molar was submerged relative to the adjacent teeth, and ankylosis was suspected. **(b)** When the patient was 6 years, 7 months old, the maxillary right first molar was erupting past the ankylosed primary second molar. **(c to e)** Nine months later, the second primary molar had submerged significantly, and the second premolar had become impacted horizontally above the roots of the primary first molar. **(f and g)** The primary second premolar was extracted, orthodontic treatment was initiated to push the maxillary first molar distally, and a maxillary Nance appliance was placed to prevent the first molar from erupting mesially.

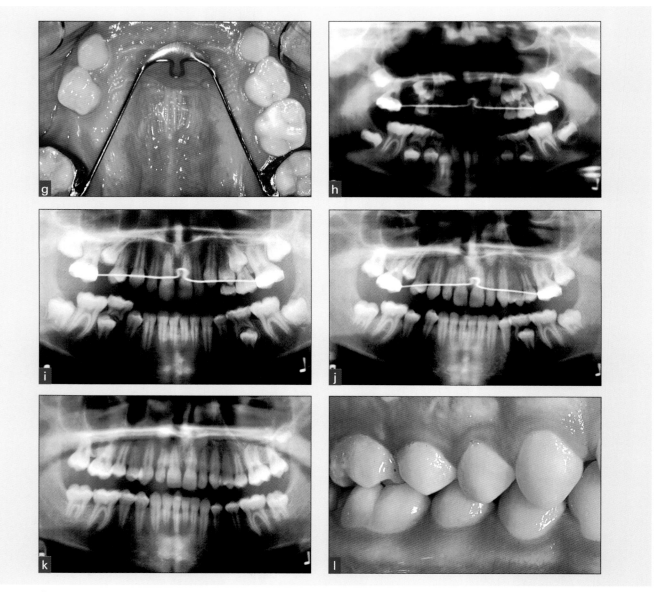

*(h to k)* Radiographs taken over the next 5 years show that the maxillary second premolar eventually erupted without any orthodontic intervention. *(l)* When the patient was 13½ years old, the second premolar had erupted completely into occlusion.

# Root Development

Impacted mandibular second premolars are often identified when the crown is fully formed but the root has just begun development. The patient in Fig 5-2 was 13 years of age and had all of her mandibular teeth, including the mandibular second molars. Although the mandibular left second premolar crown was completely calcified, the root had just begun to form. Would it be prudent to uncover the second premolar without a developed root? What would happen to the remaining root formation if the crown were uncovered and orthodontic forces were used to erupt the tooth? The literature regarding this question is not conclusive. It is the authors' opinion that early uncovering of a tooth with little to no root development could arrest further root development. Therefore, in this patient, the author (VGK) chose to wait and placed a lingual arch to maintain the position of the first molar, uncertain as to whether the second premolar would erupt. After 2 years, the premolar still had not erupted. The root had completely formed, but the tooth never erupted. Once the root had completely developed, the author (VGK) began orthodontic treatment, uncovered the crown of the tooth, and erupted the tooth into the dental arch using a Ballista spring.

# Autotransplantation

In all of the cases shown in this chapter so far, the impacted second premolars were uncovered and erupted orthodontically to achieve successful outcomes. However, in limited situations, the second premolar may be impacted in such a position that attempting to erupt the tooth orthodontically could be difficult or impossible or could jeopardize adjacent teeth and bone (see Fig 5-8b). In these situations, autotransplantation should be considered to move the tooth into its proper position (Fig 5-8). To autotransplant the second premolar, a midcrestal incision is made, and full-thickness flaps are reflected. The buccal bone is cautiously removed to locate the impacted tooth with its follicle. A crestal osteotomy is created to house the transplanted tooth (see Figs 5-8c and 5-8d). The tooth and follicle are carefully enucleated and positioned properly but in infraocclusion (see Figs 5-8e and 5-8f).

The flaps are repositioned and sutured. Orthodontic movement can be initiated in 3 months. This is an extremely difficult surgery fraught with risk of injuring the follicle and the mandibular nerve. Fortunately, in this patient there was no nerve damage or paresthesia. However, because of slight trauma to the follicle during this difficult enucleation, the tooth became ankylosed. Fortunately, this occurred after the tooth was ideally positioned orthodontically and the patient had completed her growth (see Figs 5-8q and 5-8r).

**Fig 5-8** ) **Autotransplantation of a mandibular second premolar.**

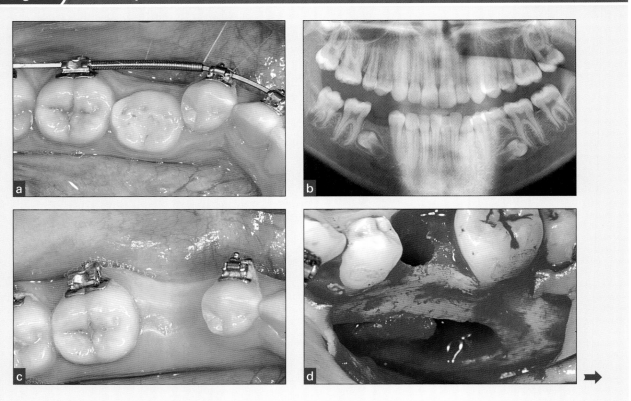

*(a and b)* This 10-year-old had two badly impacted mandibular second premolars. The primary molar was still present on the mandibular left side. The surgical plan was to uncover the mandibular right second premolar with the closed eruption technique and orthodontically upright it. The mandibular left second premolar would be surgically replanted. This tooth was so badly impacted that it would be very difficult to traditionally uncover and upright it. *(c and d)* The primary molar was extracted. Two months later, a buccal flap was reflected from the canine back to the second molar. A buccal window was made large enough to carefully enucleate the impacted second premolar, so as to not injure the follicular sac or the mandibular nerve. A second osteotomy was made on the crest of the edentulous ridge to house the transplanted tooth.

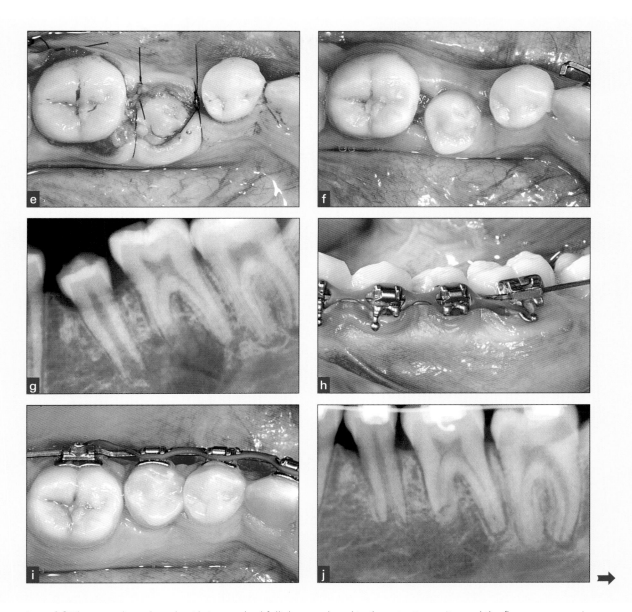

*(e and f)* The transplanted tooth with its attached follicle was placed in the osteotomy site, and the flaps were repositioned and sutured with 6-0 nylon suture. Three months later, the patient was ready to start orthodontic movement. *(g)* The radiograph shows good bone and stabilization. *(h)* After 7 months of movement, the tooth is in its proper position. *(i and j)* At the completion of orthodontic treatment, the tooth became ankylosed. Fortunately, this occurred after it was in its ideal position.

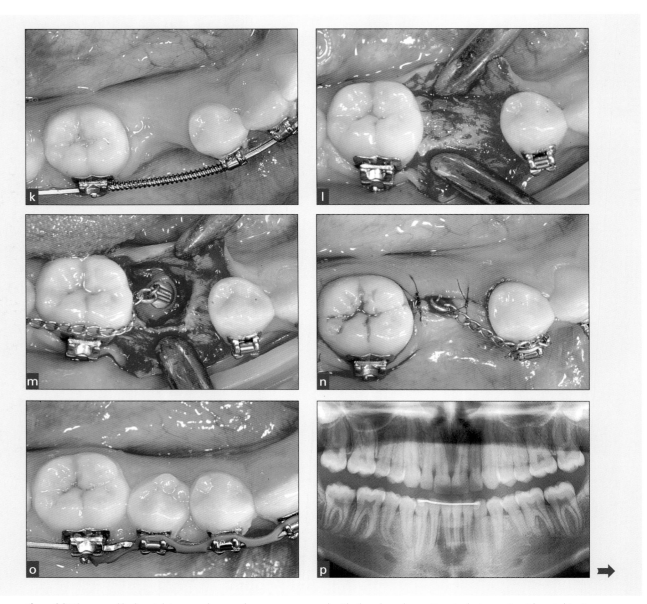

(**k and l**) The mandibular right second premolar was uncovered with the closed eruption technique. A midcrestal incision was made, and the flaps were reflected in the edentulous area. (**m and n**) Bone was removed carefully, exposing the impacted premolar. A chain was attached to the tooth, and the flaps were repositioned and sutured. The gold chain emerged through the midcrestal incision and was ligated to the bracket on the first premolar. (**o**) The tooth was orthodontically uprighted, and 10 months later it was in ideal position. (**p**) The panoramic radiograph shows both mandibular second premolars in good position.

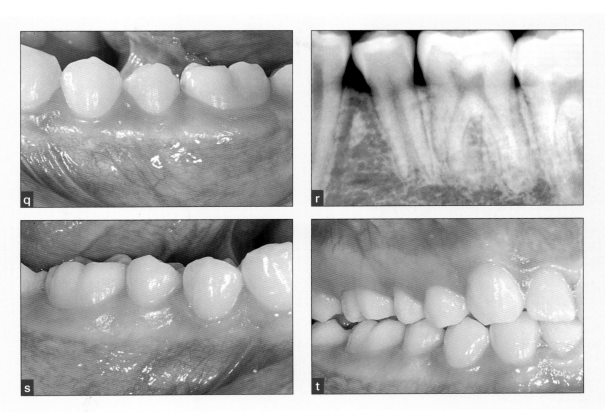

**(q and r)** Two years later, the replanted mandibular left second premolar was in good occlusion with adequate root support. **(s and t)** Similarly, the mandibular right second premolar was in good occlusion. (Courtesy of Dr David Weller [orthodontist] and Dr Jim Janakievski [periodontist], Tacoma, Washington.)

# Extraction of Impacted Premolars

It is rare that an impacted maxillary or mandibular second premolar cannot be surgically uncovered and orthodontically erupted into its proper position. However, if the surgical exposure or the orthodontic movement is deemed counterproductive for a specific patient, there is another option: extraction of the impacted premolar and closure of the edentulous space. Unfortunately, if the extraction is unilateral, there could be significant compromises to the esthetics and occlusion as a result of closing the extraction space. In these situations, it could be advantageous to utilize the anchorage provided by a strategically positioned miniscrew. This adjunct could provide sufficient anchorage to move the first and second molars mesially, thus closing the posterior edentulous space without altering the dental midline or the anterior or posterior occlusion. After the space is closed, the miniscrew can be removed.

# Recommended Reading

Abu Tair JA, Rahhal A. Tooth autotransplantation in orthodontic patients. J Contemp Dent Pract 2010;11:63–70.

Aizenbud D, Levin L, Lin S, Michtei EE. A multidisciplinary approach to the treatment of a horizontally impacted mandibular second premolar: 10-year follow-up. Orthodontics (Chic) 2011;12:48–59.

Baccetti T, Leonardi M, Giuntini V. Distally displaced premolars: A dental anomaly associated with palatally displaced canines. Am J Orthod Dentofacial Orthop 2010;138:318–322.

Becker A. An interview with Adrian Becker. World J Orthod 2004;5:277–282.

Boj JR, Hernandez M, Espasa E, Poirier C, Espanya A. Erbium laser treatment of an impacted first mandibular premolar: A case report. J Clin Pediatr Dent 2008;33:9–12.

Bokelund M, Andreasen JO, Christensen SS, Kjær I. Autotransplantation of maxillary second premolars to mandibular recipient sites where the primary second molars were impacted, predisposes for complications [epub ahead of print 3 May 2013]. Acta Odontol Scand.

Burch J, Ngan P, Hackman A. Diagnosis and treatment planning for unerupted premolars. Pediatr Dent 1994;16:89–95.

Chugh VK, Sharma VP, Tandon P, Singh GP. Treatment of an unusual crossbite with an impacted mandibular second premolar. J Clin Orthod 2008;42:341–348.

Collett AR. Conservative management of lower second premolar impaction. Aust Dent J 2000;45:279–281.

Dröschl H, Eskici A, Pilarz GF. Surgical orthodontic therapy of impacted premolars and 2d molars [in German]. Zahnartzl Prax 1977;28:74–83.

Farret MM, Farret MM, Farret AM, Hollweg H. Unusual orthodontic approach to a maxillary canine-premolar transposition and a missing lateral incisor with long-term follow-up. Am J Orthod Dentofacial Orthop 2012;142:690–697.

Fujita Y, Sorada Y, Maki K. Orthodontic treatment of a unilateral impacted mandibular canine and first premolar: A case report. Eur J Paediatr Dent 2011;12:63–66.

Halazonetis DJ. Horizontally impacted maxillary premolar and bilateral canine transposition. Am J Orthod Dentofacial Orthop 2009;135:380–389.

Kobaiashi VT, Mitomi T, Taguchi Y, Noda T. Occlusal guidance for eruption disturbance of mandibular second premolar: A report of three cases. J Clin Pediatr Dent 2003;27:101–105.

Kokich VG, Mathews DP. Surgical and orthodontic management of impacted teeth. Dent Clin North Am 1993;37:181–204.

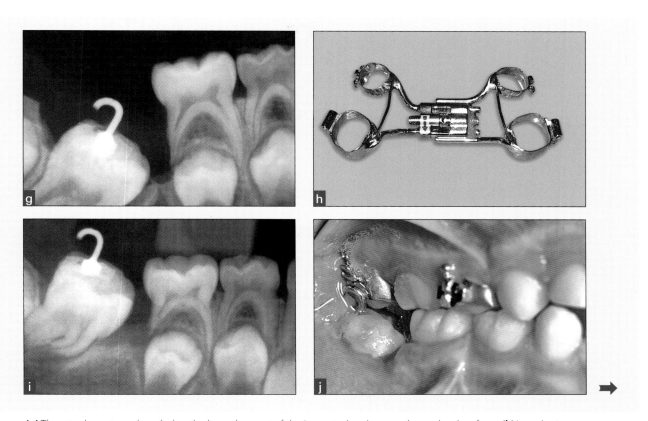

**(g)** The attachment was bonded to the buccal aspect of the impacted molar near the occlusal surface. **(h)** In order to provide enough anchorage to deliver an eruptive force to the impacted molar, a palatal expansion appliance was cemented to the maxillary permanent and primary first molars. **(i and j)** An elastic force extending from the maxillary right first molar to the hook on the mandibular first molar helped to erupt the impacted tooth in 2 months.

Impacted mandibular first molars are usually in the midalveolar position. Appropriate radiographs should be taken to confirm the location of the tooth and the root form and degree of root development. The apices of the tooth may be near the inferior border of the mandible. If they are fully developed and have significant curvatures or dilacerations, movement may be impossible. In this case, consideration may be given to luxating the tooth and elevating it to its appropriate position or slightly apical to its normal occlusal position (see Fig 6-4). It can then be bracketed and slowly moved into position. If the tooth can be uncovered, the closed eruption technique is used; however, more extensive flap reflection is needed to gain access to the apical area. Vertical incisions will facilitate

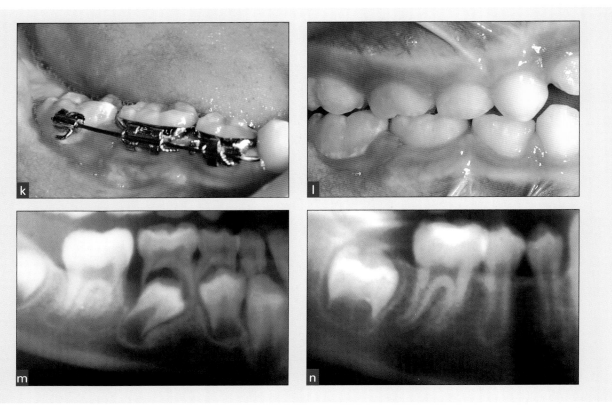

**(k)** When the hook on the mandibular first molar contacted the maxillary first molar crown, the hook was removed and brackets were placed on the three mandibular right molars, and a segmental archwire was used to complete the eruption and uprighting of the permanent first molar. **(l)** After appliance removal, the mandibular first molar was at the correct vertical level relative to the adjacent and opposing teeth. **(m)** A radiograph taken immediately after appliance removal shows that the rapid eruption of the permanent first molar had caused a change in the orientation of the developing second premolar. Also note that the root apices of the permanent first molar were still wide open after the rapid eruption process. **(n)** A panoramic radiograph taken 2 years later shows not only that the premolars erupted normally but also that the permanent first molar has erupted concomitantly with the premolars.

access for good visibility. This is imperative so that adequate bone removal can be accomplished without damaging the adjacent teeth. Care must also be taken so that the mental nerve is not damaged. When the tooth is uncovered, it is isolated and an appropriate bracket is bonded to the occlusal surface of the tooth. The bracket is custom made (see Figs 6-1f and 6-1g). It must be placed in the correct position so that the hook is not in hyperocclusion and the orthodontist has access to engage it with an elastic (see Figs 6-1i and 6-1j). The flaps are returned to their original position, and the hook is made to exit through the crestal incision for access by the orthodontist. The flaps are sutured with resorbable sutures. Tooth movement can be initiated within 1 week.

An intra-arch vertical force can be applied to the impacted tooth with a Ballista spring or elastic force attached to a distal extension of the archwire or other auxiliary appliance, such as a lingual arch. If there is inadequate space to apply intra-arch traction, an elastic force can be attached to an appliance in the opposing arch (eg, a maxillary expansion appliance [see Fig 6-1h] or a temporary anchorage device). Depending on the direction of necessary movement of the impacted molar, other auxiliary appliances such as a lingual arch in the mandibular arch or a transpalatal arch in the maxillary arch (see Fig 6-5e) can be used to stabilize the transverse and vertical positions of the anchorage units.

It is important for the orthodontist and the surgeon to discuss the details of this type of impaction before any surgery is contemplated. If it is possible to uncover the tooth and move it orthodontically, then a custom bracket must be made and its exact positioning discussed before the surgery. Good communication between the orthodontist and the surgeon will facilitate success in these difficult cases. If it is deemed that the tooth cannot be uncovered and moved without considerable risk, then extraction may be the only solution. If the tooth can be luxated and positioned occlusally, then the surgeon and the orthodontist must discuss the exact location at which it will be positioned at surgery and how the tooth will be bracketed and stabilized.

## Second Molars

Mandibular second molars are usually impacted in the midalveolar region. When they are angulated mesially and locked under the first molar (Fig 6-2), they will need to be uncovered and left uncovered so that the orthodontist can apply appropriate mechanics to erupt the tooth (Figs 6-2d and 6-2e). The closed eruption technique, as demonstrated with the case of the first molar (see Fig 6-1), cannot be used. A modification of this technique with the flap design must be employed.

A gingivectomy is not adequate to uncover enough of the buccal surface of the mandibular second molar. There is usually a shallow vestibule in this location and a minimal amount of gingiva. The best access can be achieved with a conservative lingual flap. The buccal needs to be apically positioned, so vertical incisions are necessary (see Fig 6-2e). This flap design will allow the surgeon access for adequate bone removal. It will also facilitate apical positioning of the buccal and lingual flaps so that the tooth is left exposed for easy bracketing and appropriate orthodontic mechanics. A dressing is placed on the buccal surface to avoid hypertrophy so that the tooth stays uncovered. In 2 weeks, the tooth can be bracketed and tooth movement can be initiated.

Impacted molars present special orthodontic challenges in terms of anchorage and the space available to apply vertical force. Almost always, the best option for impacted molars is to have the tooth exposed enough so that a bracket or tube can be bonded to the buccal surface (see Fig 6-2). Among other advantages, this allows direct visualization of tooth position and easy modification of force vectors. If only partial exposure can be achieved or if the surface exposed is not the buccal, then an attachment (see Figs 6-1f and 6-1g) must be placed on any available surface. Its position will have to be periodically changed to accomplish the desired tooth movement.

## Fig 6-2  Impacted mandibular left second molar.

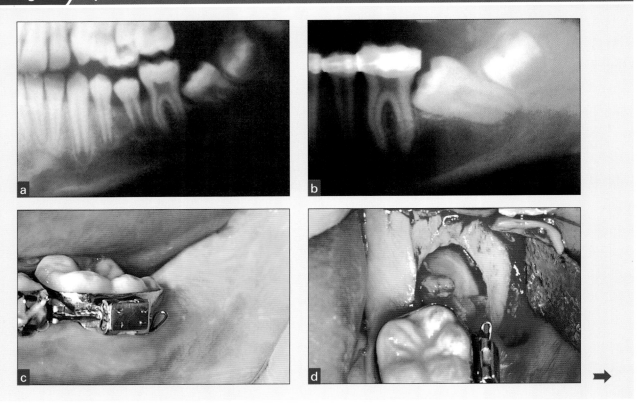

*(a)* This adolescent boy was initially referred for orthodontic treatment at 11 years of age. *(b)* Orthodontic treatment was begun, and after 1 year a radiograph was taken to determine why the mandibular left second molar had not erupted. The radiograph showed that the second molar had tipped mesially during root development and was incapable of erupting. *(c)* The intraoral photograph at that time shows that the crown of the tooth was not visible. *(d)* A midcrestal incision was made, and full-thickness flaps were reflected. The occlusal surface of the impacted tooth was visible, but the buccal and lingual aspects were completely covered with bone.

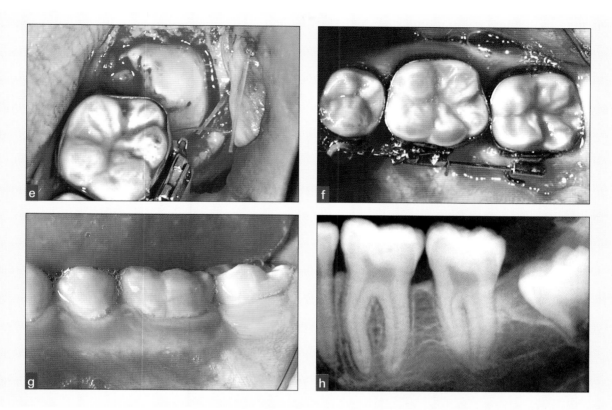

(e) Bone removal was accomplished to expose the entire buccal aspect of the crown, and the buccal flap was positioned apically so that the crown would remain uncovered. This would permit complete access to the crown and simplify the uprighting process for the orthodontist. Initially, a bracket was bonded to the buccal surface of the crown, and a flexible wire was used to upright the tooth. (f) Eventually, a band was cemented to the crown to complete the uprighting process. (g) After appliance removal, the intraoral photograph shows that the zone of gingiva labial to the second molar has been maintained. (h) The periapical radiograph taken after orthodontic treatment shows that the bone support on the distal of the first molar and mesial of the second molar has been improved substantially during the orthodontic uprighting. Because the uprighting of the second molar was successful, the third molar was scheduled to be extracted following orthodontic treatment.

**Fig 6-3** ) **Exposure and eruption of impacted mandibular second molars.**

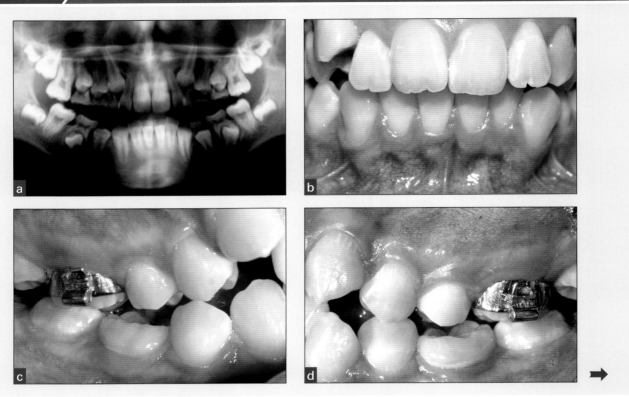

This adolescent patient was referred for correction of a Class III malocclusion. **(a)** The panoramic radiograph shows ectopically positioned mandibular second premolars and congenitally missing mandibular third molars. **(b to d)** The intraoral photographs show normal overjet and overbite and bilateral Class III molar relationships. The plan was to extract the mandibular second premolars because of their poor positioning and to provide space for correction of the arch length deficiency. Despite the creation of adequate space in the posterior part of the arch, the mandibular second molars failed to erupt. Both second molars were then surgically exposed. Buccal and lingual flaps were reflected, and bone was removed from the occlusal of the molars. In addition, some buccal and lingual bone was removed to uncover the height of contour. The flaps were apically positioned with resorbable sutures, and a dressing was placed.

If the impacted molar has been moved a large distance, special retention procedures should be used (Fig 6-3). Frequently, a fixed spiral wire is bonded to the buccal surfaces of the adjacent teeth to prevent space reopening (see Figs 6-3h to 6-3j). Removable retainers are also used to prevent buccal, lingual, or vertical movement of the previously impacted tooth.

Impacted mandibular second molars can also be moved surgically. If the tooth is submerged vertically or is mesially impacted, surgical positioning may be considered (Fig 6-4). The treatment is similar to that used with the mandibular first molar. Coordination between the surgeon and the orthodontist is imperative to discuss the position of the tooth, means of stabilizing the tooth at surgery, and type of bracket needed.

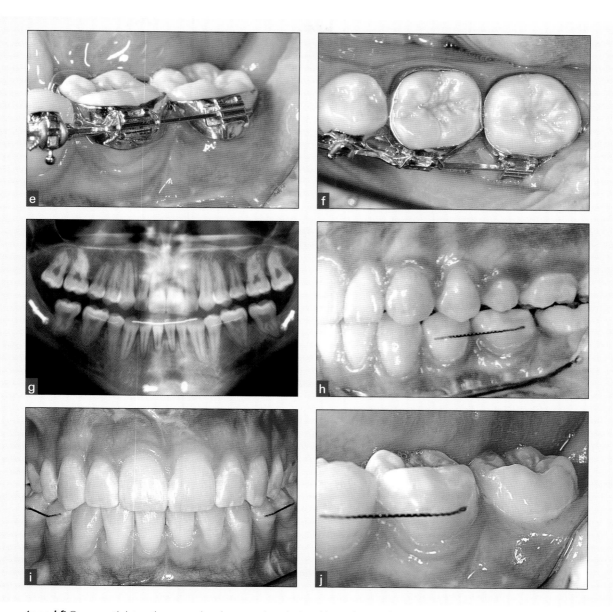

(e and f) One month later, the second molars were banded and brought into the arch. (g) The posttreatment radiograph shows the surgical plates used to fixate the mandible and the fixed lingual retainer. (h and i) The posttreatment photographs show normal overjet and overbite and Class I canine and Class III molar relationships. (j) Twisted spiral wires were bonded to the buccal surfaces of the first premolars and first molars to prevent reopening of the extraction spaces.

## Fig 6-4 Surgical uprighting of an impacted mandibular left second molar.

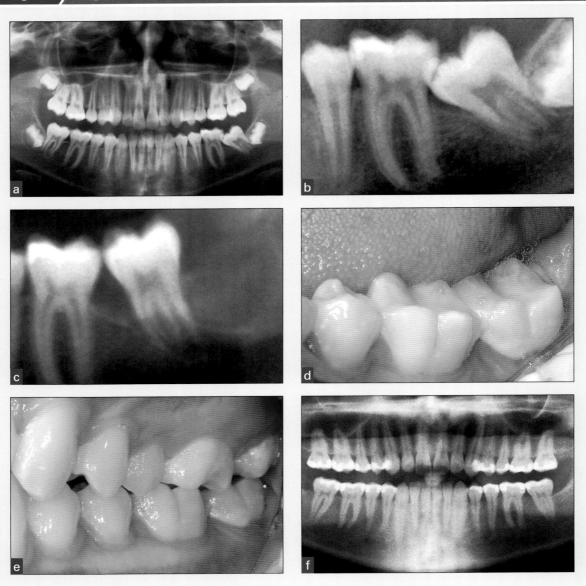

(a) All of this 12 year-old boy's permanent teeth had erupted except for the mandibular left second molar. (b) This tooth was tipped mesially and impacted apical to the height of contour of the first molar. (c) The boy had a normal Angle Class I malocclusion with no apparent need for orthodontic treatment, so instead of placing brackets and bands on the teeth to facilitate orthodontic uprighting of the second molar, the tooth was surgically uprighted and the third molar was extracted at the same time. (d) One year later, the intraoral photograph shows that the second molar has maintained its proper position relative to the adjacent first molar. (e and f) The 5-year follow-up photograph and radiograph show good bone support and root alignment. (Orthodontics courtesy of Dr Doug Knight, Tacoma, Washington.)

**Fig 6-5** ) **Impacted maxillary left first and second molars.**

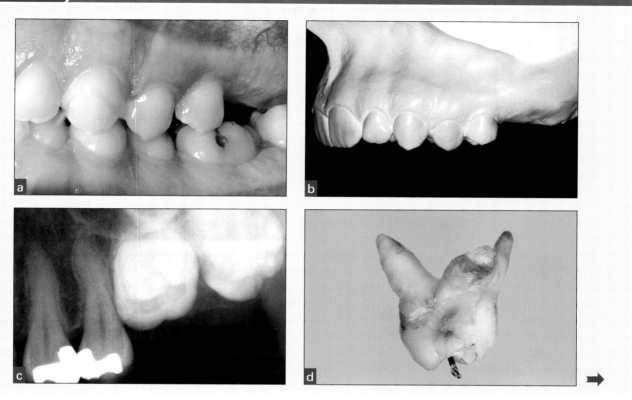

(a to c) The maxillary left first and second molars were impacted in the alveolus of this adult female. As a result, the mandibular first and second molars had overerupted. The initial plan was to level the mandibular arch orthodontically, uncover both maxillary molars, and place an attachment on the second molar to erupt it into position first. However, the second molar would not move, even with luxation by the surgeon. (d) Therefore, the second molar was extracted. Note the divergent roots of the maxillary second molar, which could have slowed and prevented the second molar from erupting properly.

# Maxillary Molars

Note that maxillary molars can also become impacted. Figure 6-5 illustrates a case in which the maxillary first and second molars were impacted in an adult.

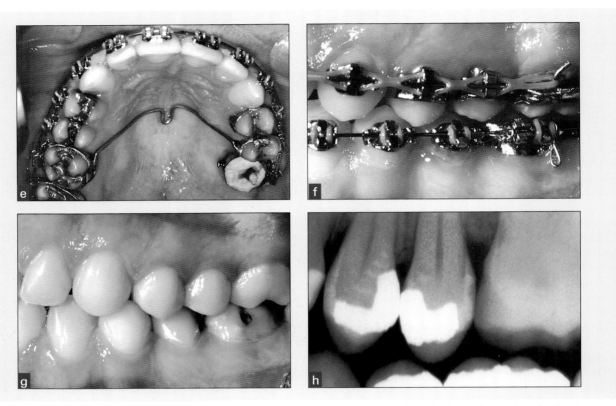

**(e)** Subsequently, the first molar was luxated by the surgeon, a band was cemented on the first molar, and a palatal arch was constructed from the right first molar to the left second premolar to aid in providing anchorage to erupt the first molar. **(f)** A flexible wire was used to erupt the first molar into occlusion. **(g and h)** An intraoral photograph and radiograph taken 4 years after orthodontic treatment show that the eruption of the first molar was successful and that the bone levels between the second premolar and the first molar are normal.

# Recommended Reading

Barberia-Leache E, Suarez-Clúa MC, Saavedra-Ontiveros D. Ectopic eruption of the maxillary first permanent molar: Characteristics and occurrence in growing children. Angle Orthod 2005;75:610–615.

Bokelund M, Andreasen JO, Christensen SS, Kjær I. Autotransplantation of maxillary second premolars to mandibular recipient sites where the primary second molars were impacted, predisposes for complications [epub ahead of print 3 May 2013]. Acta Odontol Scand.

Cassetta M, Altieri F, Di Mambro A, Galluccio G, Barbato E. Impaction of permanent mandibular second molar: A retrospective study. Med Oral Patol Oral Cir Bucal 2013;18:e564–e568.

De Massiac G. Orthodontic repositioning technic of impacted lower 2nd molars [in French]. Rev Stomatol Chir Maxillofac 1994;95:38–43.

Farronato G, Giannini L, Galbiati G, Consonni D, Maspero C. Spontaneous eruption of impacted second molars. Prog Orthod 2011;12:119–125.

Ferro F, Funiciello G, Perillo L, Chiodini P. Mandibular lip bumper treatment and second molar eruption disturbances. Am J Orthod Dentofacial Orthop 2011;139:622–627.

Fu PS, Wang JC, Chen CH, Huang TK, Tseng CH, Hung CC. Management of unilaterally deep impacted first, second, and third mandibular molars. Angle Orthod 2012;82:565–571.

Fu PS, Wang JC, Wu YM, et al. Impacted mandibular second molars. Angle Orthod 2012;82:670–675.

Fujita T, Shirakura M, Hayashi H, Tsuka Y, Fujii E, Tanne K. Uprighting of severely impacted mandibular second molars: A case report. Aust Orthod J 2012;28:258–264.

Hegde S, Munshi AK. Management of an impacted, dilacerated mandibular left permanent first molar: A case report. Quintessence Int 2001;32:235–237.

Hennessy J, Al-Awadhi EA, Dwyer LO, Leith R. Treatment of ectopic first permanent molar teeth. Dent Update 2012;39:656–658,660–661.

Jerrold TL. Bilateral impactions of mandibular first, second, and third molars. Am J Orthod 1966;52:190–201.

Kennedy DB. Management of an ectopically erupting permanent mandibular molar: A case report. Pediatr Dent 2008;30:63–65.

Kokich VG, Mathews DP. Surgical and orthodontic management of impacted teeth. Dent Clin North Am 1993;37:181–204.

Lau CK, Whang CZ, Bister D. Orthodontic uprighting of severely impacted mandibular second molars. Am J Orthod Dentofacial Orthop 2013;143:116–124.

Majourau A, Norton LA. Uprighting impacted second molars with segmented springs. Am J Orthod Dentofacial Orthop 1995;107:235–238.

Park JH, Tai K, Iida S. Unilateral delayed eruption of a mandibular permanent canine and the maxillary first and second molars, and agenesis of the maxillary third molar. Am J Orthod Dentofacial Orthop 2013;143:134–139.

Proff P, Bayerlein T, Fanghänel J, Allegrini S Jr, Gedrange T. Morphological and clinical considerations of first and second permanent molar eruption disorders. Ann Anat 2006;188:353–361.

Reddy SK, Uloopi KS, Vinay C, Subba Reddy VV. Orthodontic uprighting of impacted mandibular permanent second molar: A case report. J Indian Soc Pedod Prev Dent 2008;26:29–31.

Resch D. Clinical management of unilaterally impacted mandibular first and second molars. J Clin Orthod 2003;37:162–164.

Rizzatto SM, de Menezes LM, do Rego MV, Thiesen G, de Araujo VP, Freitas MP. Maxillary first permanent molar impaction. A conservative treatment approach. J Clin Pediatr Dent 2005;30:169–173.

Seehra J, Winchester L, DiBiase AT, Cobourne MT. Orthodontic management of ectopic maxillary first permanent molars: A case report. Aust Orthod J 2011;27:57–62.

Shapiro Y, Finkelstein T, Shpack N, Lai YH, Kuftinec MM, Vardimon A. Mandibular second molar impaction. I. Genetic traits and characteristics. Am J Orthod Dentofacial Orthop 2011;140:32–37.

Smith CP, Al-Awadhi EA, Garvey MT. An atypical presentation of mechanical failure of eruption of a mandibular permanent molar: Diagnosis and treatment case report. Eur Arch Paediatr Dent 2012;13:152–156.

Vedtofte H, Andreasen JO, Kjær I. Arrested eruption of the permanent lower second molar. Eur J Orthod 1999;21:31–40.

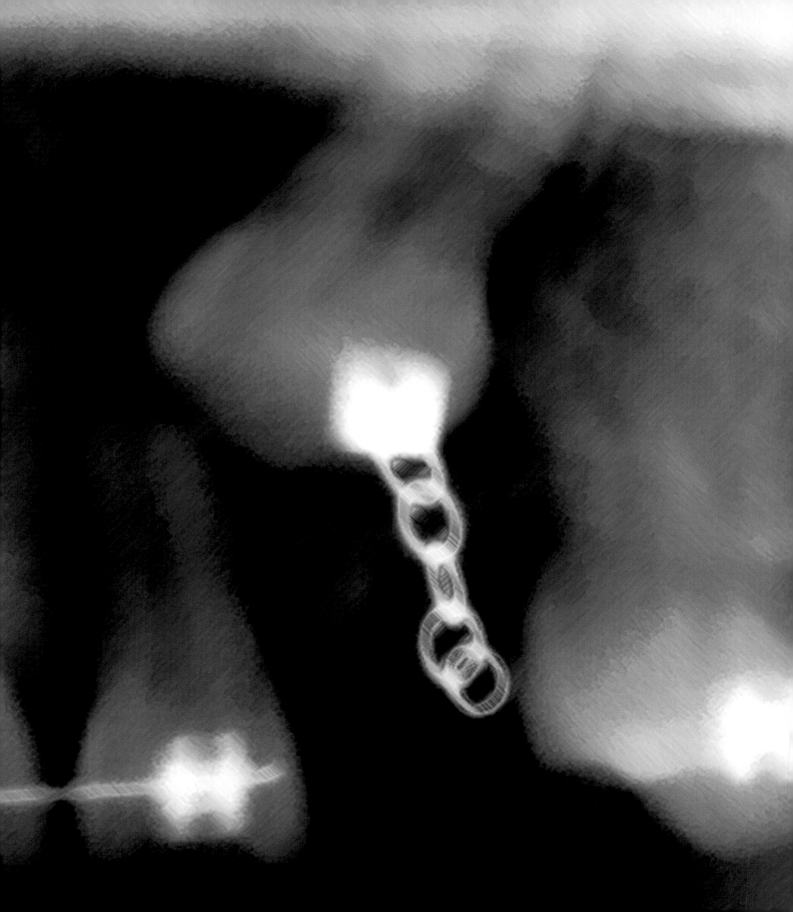

# Complications and Adverse Sequelae

## 7

The treatment of impacted teeth in adolescents and adults can be fraught with many different problems. Most of these problems are related to improper diagnosis, inappropriate surgery, or incorrect orthodontic mechanics. These problems have been discussed within each chapter.

Any one of these problems can lead to serious sequelae in the treatment of an impacted tooth. A combination of factors can lead to periodontal bone loss (Figs 7-1 to 7-3), tooth loss (Figs 7-4 to 7-6), or devastating esthetic results that may be difficult to correct (Fig 7-7). The purpose of this chapter is to help the clinician avoid these pitfalls. Orthodontists know that inappropriate treatment of impacted teeth is one of the leading causes of adverse litigation in orthodontics. However, all of these pitfalls are avoidable with proper diagnosis, surgery, and orthodontic treatment.

In this chapter, the authors share their most important "lessons learned" from 40 years of treating impacted teeth.

**Fig 7-1** Improper orthodontic mechanics resulting in bone loss.

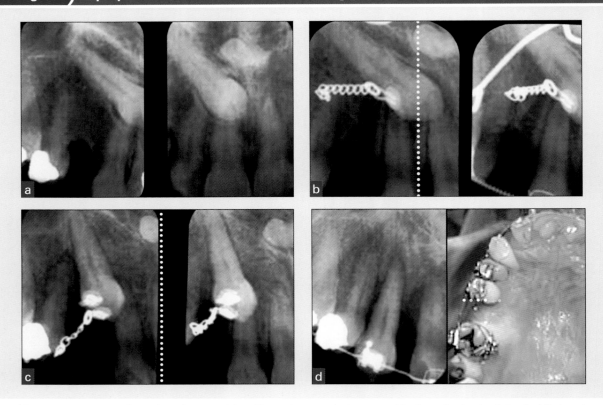

This case was sent to the authors for an opinion. The patient was being treated in the orthodontic clinic of a US dental school. *(a)* The maxillary right canine in this 49-year-old woman was impacted palatally. *(b and c)* The tooth was uncovered, a chain was bonded to the lingual surface, the flap was repositioned, and the tooth was being pulled in a distal direction underneath the flap. *(d)* The orthodontic resident who was treating this patient stated that the time interval between *(a)* and *(d)* was 3.5 years. The concern of the orthodontic resident was the significant bone loss that had occurred on the distal of the left lateral incisor and mesial, distal, and palatal aspects of the maxillary right canine. **Lesson:** Autonomous eruption or appropriate force direction during the orthodontics could have prevented this advanced bone loss on the lateral incisor, canine, and premolar.

### Fig 7-2 ) Poorly executed surgery and orthodontics resulting in advanced bone loss.

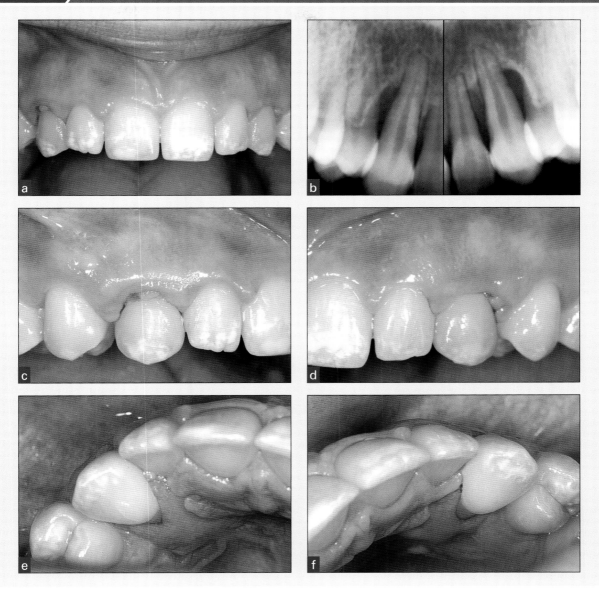

(a to f) This adolescent girl was referred to the authors after orthodontic treatment for an opinion about the prognosis and possible treatment of the maxillary right and left canines and lateral incisors. The canines were originally impacted in the palate and surgically uncovered at least two times. Each time, they were immediately chained and dragged toward the edentulous area. The probing depths were 5 to 9 mm around the lateral incisors and canines. There was also significant mobility of these teeth. **Lesson:** Proper surgery and autonomous eruption would have prevented this disastrous bone loss.

## Fig 7-3 ) Injudicious surgery resulting in extensive bone loss and devitalization of the canine.

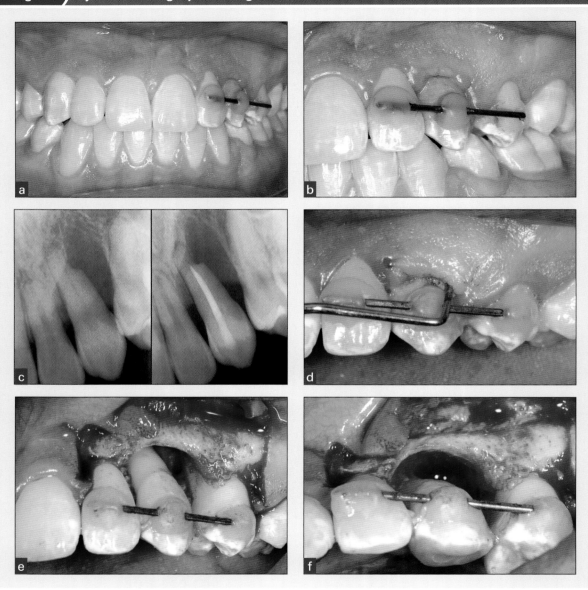

This adolescent boy was referred to the authors after orthodontic treatment for an opinion regarding the prognosis of the maxillary left lateral incisor and canine. The canine was palatally impacted and uncovered three times. *(a and b)* After orthodontics, the canine was extremely mobile, and a wire splint was bonded to the adjacent teeth to stabilize the tooth. *(c)* The radiograph shows the extensive bone loss around the canine. The canine pulp was nonvital, so root canal therapy was completed. *(d)* Six months after endodontic therapy, the probing depths on the labial and distal surfaces were still 10 mm. *(e and f)* Surgical exposure of the area revealed that a well-type osseous defect extended circumferentially around the canine root. **Lesson:** Minimal surgery to expose the crown of the impacted canine and autonomous eruption or better orthodontic mechanics could have prevented this severe bone loss on the premolar and canine.

## Fig 7-4 ) Ligation of a palatally impacted maxillary left canine resulting in loss of the tooth.

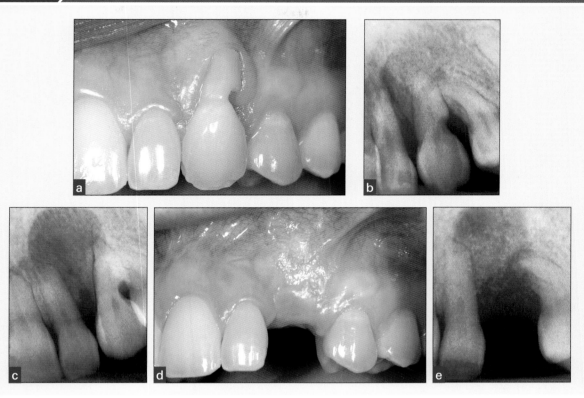

**(a)** This adolescent girl was referred to the periodontist for a gingival graft to cover the exposed root of the maxillary left canine. The history of this situation revealed that the left canine was palatally impacted. It had been uncovered, ligated, and moved orthodontically into the dental arch. However, severe gingival recession was evident after appliance removal. The recession extended to the level of the root apex. **(b and c)** The radiographs show that there was significant inflammatory resorption on the distal root surface. The pulp of the canine was nonvital. In addition, there was a large periodontal-endodontic radiolucency. **(d and e)** This hopeless situation resulted in the loss of the previously impacted maxillary left canine. **Lesson:** Do not ligate impacted teeth. Use very judicious bone removal during the uncovering.

**Fig 7-5** ) **Ligation of the maxillary right canine resulting in loss of teeth.**

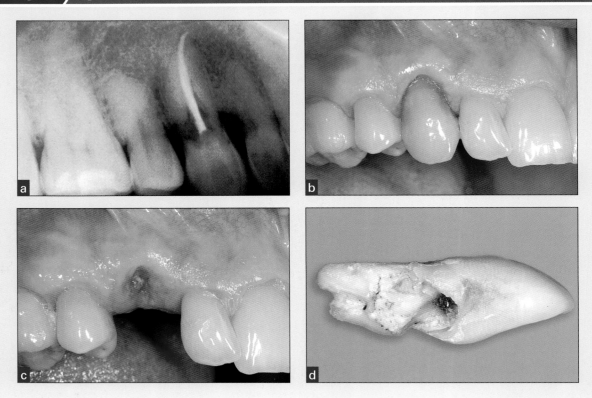

This 40-year-old man had undergone orthodontic treatment as a child. The maxillary right canine had been impacted palatally. The tooth had been uncovered and a ligature wire lasso placed around the tooth. After completion of orthodontic treatment, some cervical resorption was evident and root canal therapy was necessary because of loss of pulpal vitality. *(a and b)* Twenty-five years later, further resorption of the lateral and canine roots was evident. *(c)* The patient delayed any treatment, and 1 year later the canine crown fractured, leaving the root remaining within the alveolus. *(d)* Subsequently, the lateral incisor was also extracted due to the extensive cervical root resorption. **Lesson:** The ligated canine was pulled into the root of the lateral incisor, causing root resorption and ultimate loss of both teeth. Better force mechanics could have prevented the loss of the lateral incisor.

**Fig 7-6** ) **Late diagnosis of an impacted maxillary right canine resulting in significant root resorption.**

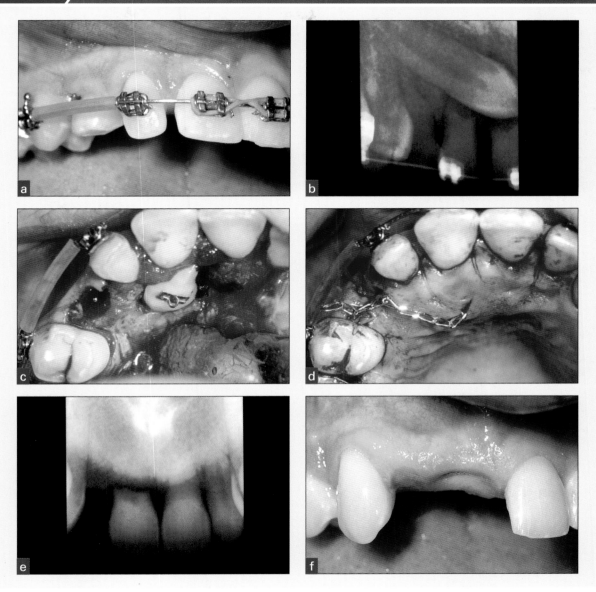

This patient was referred to a periodontist for implant replacement of the maxillary right central and lateral incisors. *(a and b)* As evident in the photographic and radiographic history of this patient, the maxillary right canine was palatally impacted and had caused significant resorption of the right central and lateral incisors. *(c and d)* The canine was uncovered, a chain was attached, and the flap was repositioned. *(e and f)* Subsequent movement of the canine in a lateral and occlusal direction caused further resorption of the lateral and central incisor roots, resulting in the loss of both teeth after orthodontic treatment. **Lesson:** Early diagnosis could have prevented this devastating root resorption. Once the canine is misdirected and begins resorbing the adjacent root, it should be uncovered and moved away from the resorbing roots.

**Fig 7-7** Failed attempt at autotransplantation resulting in loss of teeth and extensive defect.

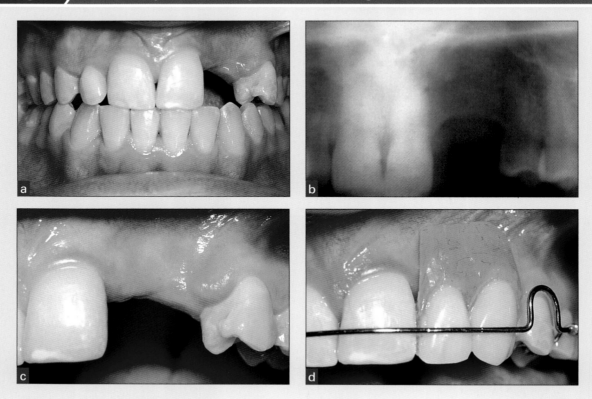

*(a to d)* This patient was referred to a periodontist for implant replacement of the maxillary left lateral incisor and canine. Apparently the canine was palatally impacted and a surgeon had attempted autotransplantation of the canine into the alveolar ridge. However, the procedure failed, resulting in loss of the lateral incisor and canine and leaving a significant labial and vertical alveolar defect. **Lesson:** Palatally impacted canines have a very high success rate when uncovered and moved properly. Autotransplantation of a palatally impacted canine into a deficient ridge is very risky.

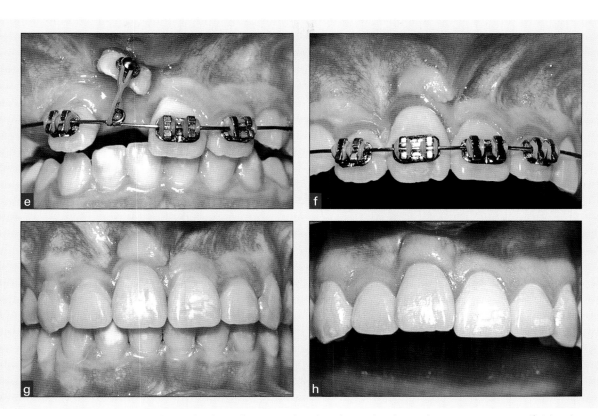

**(e)** After the tissue had healed, an orthodontic force was placed on the tooth to begin the eruption process. **(f)** A bracket was eventually placed on the right central incisor to complete the tooth positioning. **(g)** At the completion of orthodontic treatment, the incisal edge of the right central incisor was even with that of the left central incisor. There was a gingival margin discrepancy between the two central incisors that was corrected with a gingivectomy on the left central incisor. **(h)** However, after 2 years, the right central incisor had migrated apically. **Lesson:** Uncover this type of impaction with the closed eruption technique or consider surgical replantation.

**Fig 7-10** | **Improper surgery of an impacted maxillary left central incisor resulting in gingival recession.**

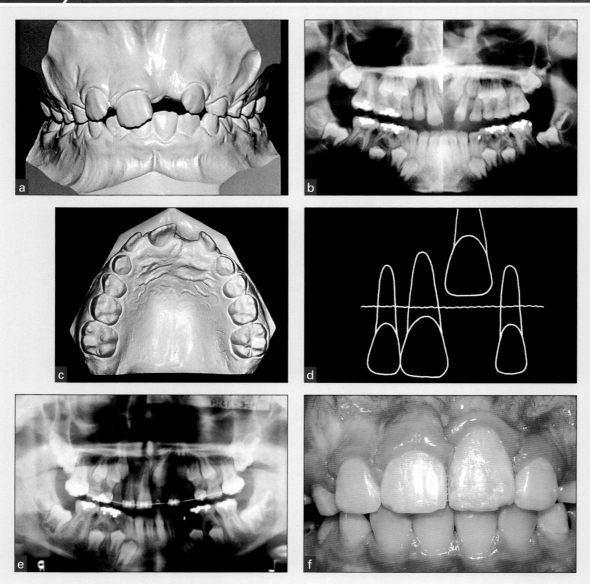

*(a to d)* This 9-year-old boy had an impacted maxillary left central incisor that was located near the middle of the alveolus and above the mucogingival junction. *(e)* Orthodontic brackets were placed on the adjacent incisors, and the central incisor was exposed by making a fenestration through the mucosa. The tooth was erupted into the dental arch. *(f)* After bracket removal, there was a significant discrepancy in clinical crown lengths between the two central incisors. In addition, the rolled labial gingival margin over the left central incisor is readily apparent. **Lesson:** Uncover this type of impacted central incisor with the closed eruption technique.

**Fig 7-11** ) **Labially impacted maxillary left canine uncovered with the closed eruption technique.**

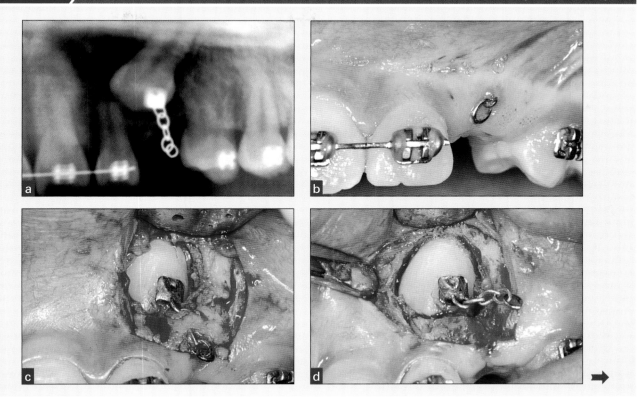

*(a and b)* This adolescent girl had a labially impacted maxillary left canine that had been uncovered with the closed erup-tion technique. The tooth had made some progress in moving coronally but suddenly stopped responding to orthodon-tic forces. *(c)* The tooth was re-uncovered with an apically positioned flap, and it was noted that bone had grown over the chain. *(d)* Bone was removed from the chain, and further bone removal was accomplished to expose more of the crown.

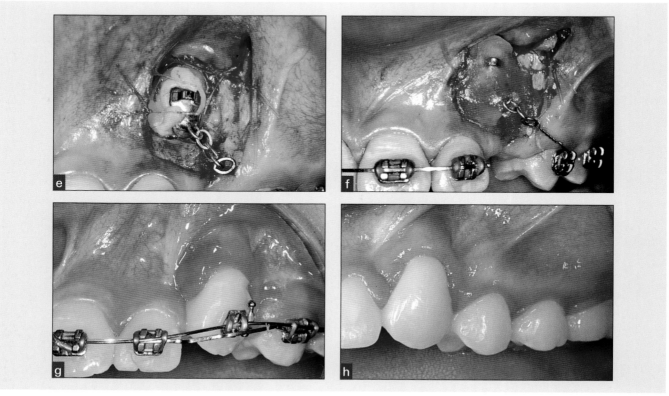

*(e and f)* The flap was apically positioned, exposing the crown of the tooth, and a dressing was placed over the exposed tooth. *(g and h)* The tooth was eventually moved successfully into the dental arch. **Lesson:** Because of the angle of this ectopically positioned canine, a modified apically positioned flap would allow better access and orthodontic mechanics to move it successfully. It would also reduce the risk of root resorption on the lateral incisor.

## Fig 7-12 Recession on a labially impacted and ectopically positioned mandibular left canine.

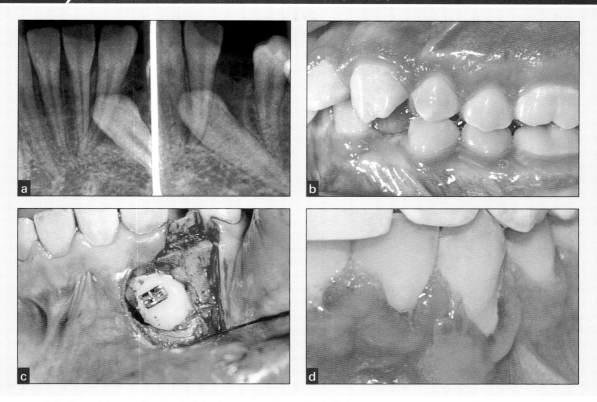

(a and b) This adolescent boy had a labially impacted mandibular left canine that was ectopically positioned over the root of the left lateral incisor. (c) A flap was elevated from the edentulous area. Bone was removed from the impacted tooth, exposing two-thirds of the crown, and the flap was apically positioned. (d) After orthodontic treatment was completed, the canine showed evidence of inflammation and moderate gingival recession. **Lesson:** Avoiding recession on this type of impaction is difficult. Sometimes the area can be pregrafted with a free gingival graft. Repair of this type of recession with a connective tissue graft is very predictable. The modified apically positioned flap is also being tested for this type of impaction to see if spontaneous eruption will occur with minimal recession.

**Fig 7-13** | **Improper uncovering and orthodontic mechanics resulting in lack of movement of the right canine.**

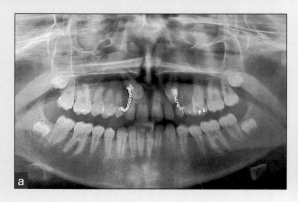 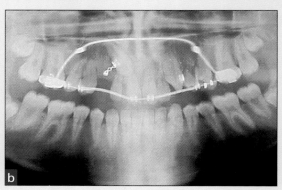

An orthodontist emailed these radiographs to the authors for an opinion. *(a)* Both maxillary canines were impacted and were uncovered using the closed eruption technique. The left canine was located in the middle of the alveolus between the roots of the lateral incisor and premolar. *(b)* After 12 months, the orthodontic force had successfully moved the left canine coronally. However, the orthodontist's concern was the lack of movement of the right canine, which was originally located labial to the lateral incisor. In spite of significant force and the evident distortion of the maxillary archwire, the right canine had not moved. **Lesson:** This ectopically positioned impacted labial canine needed to be left uncovered with a modified apically positioned flap. Then appropriate orthodontic mechanics would have erupted it easily without damaging the anchorage teeth.

# Index

Page numbers followed by "f" denote figures

## A

Adverse sequelae
    bone loss, 155, 156f–158f
    esthetic-related, 155
    maxillary central incisor impaction, 168f
    overview of, 155
    tooth loss, 155, 159f–161f
Alveolus, maxillary central incisor impaction in, 4f
Ankylosis
    palatally impacted maxillary canines and, 87, 92
    premolar impaction affected by, 130, 131f–132f
Apically positioned flap
    labially impacted maxillary canines uncovered with, 28, 31f–35f, 37, 41, 62f, 63, 164f–165f
    mandibular canine impaction uncovered with, 106, 108
    mandibular second molar impaction uncovered with, 145
    maxillary central incisor impaction uncovered with, 6, 7f–10f, 23–24, 166f–167f
    problems associated with, 6, 23–24
    with resorbable sutures, 35f
Arch length discrepancy, 66, 66f
Archwire, 82f, 88
Autotransplantation
    mandibular second premolar impaction treated with, 133, 134f–137f
    tooth loss secondary to failure of, 162f

## B

Ballista loop/spring, 13f, 23, 37f, 51, 105, 105f, 126, 129
Barricaid dressing, 43f, 47f
Bone loss, 155, 156f–158f
Bracket(s)
    mandibular canine impaction treated with, 105, 108
    maxillary central incisor impaction treated with, 5
Bracket and chain, for uncovering labially impacted maxillary canines, 52f–54f
Buccal object rule, 44, 46f, 94f

**C**

Canines. *See* Labially impacted maxillary canines; Mandibular canine impaction; Palatally impacted maxillary canines.
Cementoenamel junction, 48, 65
Cervical headgear, 72
Cleat
   and chain, for uncovering labially impacted maxillary canine, 42f–44f, 62f
   for uncovering palatally impacted maxillary canine, 78, 78f
Closed eruption technique
   description of, 72
   labially impacted maxillary canines uncovered with, 28, 36f–37f, 38, 48, 60, 63, 169f–170f
   mandibular canine impaction uncovered with, 103–104
   maxillary central incisor impaction uncovered with, 11–19, 12f–19f
   palatally impacted maxillary canines uncovered with, 72–74
   premolar impaction uncovered with, 119–125, 120f–125f
   root resorption concerns, 74
   tooth attachment methods, 60
Complex palatally impacted maxillary canines
   ankylosis of, 87, 92
   definition of, 75
   elastomeric chain for uncovering of, 81f–82f
   full-thickness flap for uncovering of, 87, 88f–89f
Complications. *See* Adverse sequelae.
Cone beam computed tomography, of labially impacted maxillary canines, 44, 60, 61f
Crestal osteotomy, 133

**D**

Dentigerous cyst, 4

**E**

Early diagnosis, 163
Ectopic impactions
   labially impacted maxillary canines
      adverse sequelae involving, 172f
      apically positioned flap for, 38, 41, 51, 164f–165f
      lateral incisor root angulation considerations, 65
      modified flap design for uncovering of, 45, 46f–47f
      orthodontics for, 51–53
      over maxillary central incisor, 59
   mandibular canines
      description of, 103
      illustration of, 106f–107f, 109f–110f
      recession on, 171f
   mandibular second premolar, 120f–121f
Elastomeric chain
   tooth movement facilitated using, 126

   for uncovering palatally impacted maxillary canine, 81f–82f
Excisional uncovering
   of impacted maxillary central incisors, 5, 6f, 23
   of labially impacted maxillary canines, 28, 29f–30f
Extraction
   of impacted premolars, 138
   of labially impacted maxillary canines, 65, 66f–67f

**F**

First molar impaction, 141–145, 142f–144f
Full-thickness flaps
   illustration of, 61f
   mandibular canines uncovered with, 111f–112f
   palatally impacted maxillary canines uncovered with, 77, 79f–80f, 83f–89f
   premolar impaction uncovered with, 119

**G**

Gingival graft, 63, 111
Gingival recession, 63, 168f
Gingivectomy
   labially impacted maxillary canines uncovered with, 30f
   maxillary central incisor impaction uncovered with, 5, 6f, 23
   problems associated with, 23
Gold chain, for erupting premolar impaction, 119, 122f

**H**

Horizontal impactions
   labially impacted maxillary canines, 48, 49f
   mandibular canine, 108, 109f–110f
   mandibular second premolar, 116f
   maxillary central incisor
      apically positioned flap for, 7f–8f, 166f–167f
      closed eruption technique for, 18f–19f
      relapse of, 166f–167f
      surgical replantation of, 20f–22f

**I**

Incisors. *See* Lateral incisor; Maxillary central incisor impaction.

**L**

Labially impacted maxillary canines
   adjacent lateral incisor considerations, 59
   apical, nondisplaced impaction, 48, 49f–50f
   arch length discrepancy, 66, 66f
   auxiliary labial bow for movement of, 58

coronal, nondisplaced impaction, 30f, 48
crown length discrepancies, 65
crown position
    labiolingual, 37
    mesiodistal, 38
direction of tooth movement, 64–65
ectopic
    apically positioned flap for, 38, 41, 51,
        164f–165f
    lateral incisor root angulation
        considerations, 65
    modified flap design for uncovering of,
        45, 46f–47f
    orthodontics for, 51–53
    over maxillary central incisor, 59
esthetics of, 63
etiology of, 28
extraction of, 65, 66f–67f
gingiva amount in area of, 38
gingival recession associated with, 63
horizontal, 48, 49f
illustration of, 29f
imaging of, 60, 61f–62f
lack of tooth movement, 63–64, 172f
lateral incisor and, 61f–62f, 65
location determinations for, 44, 46f
midalveolar, high, nondisplaced impaction
    apically positioned flap for, 51
    orthodontics for, 51
    uncovering of, 50
near lateral incisor, 61f–62f
orthodontic mechanics for
    anchorage considerations, 53
    challenges, 55, 55f–59f, 58–59
    ectopic impaction, 51–53, 52f–54f
    midalveolar impaction, 51
prevalence of, 27
relapse and recession on, 164f–165f
root resorption, 39f–41f, 58f–59f, 60, 64
self-correction of, 28
slightly, 34f–35f
spontaneous eruption of, 46f–47f
surgery for
    buccal object rule, 44, 46f
    cone beam computed tomography
        before, 44, 60, 61f
    location determinations before, 44
tooth movement
    direction of, 64–65
    extraction versus, 66, 66f–67f
    lack of, 63–64, 172f
uncovering of
    adverse sequelae, 172f
    apically positioned flap for, 28, 31f–35f,
        37–38, 51, 62f, 63, 164f–165f
    bracket and chain for, 52f–54f
    cleat and chain for, 42f–44f, 62f
    closed eruption technique for, 28, 36f–37f,
        38, 48, 60, 63, 169f–170f
    criteria for selecting method for, 37–38
    excisional, 28, 29f–30f
    gingivectomy for, 30f
    pin for, 36f–37f

Lateral incisor
    labially impacted maxillary canine near the
        apex of, 61f–62f
    positioning of, 65
Ligation, of palatally impacted maxillary
    canines, 159f–160f


**M**
Mandibular canine impaction
    brackets for, 108
    ectopic
        description of, 103
        illustration of, 106f–107f, 109f–110f
        recession on, 171f
    horizontal, 108, 109f–110f
    labial
        description of, 103
        ectopic positioning of, 106, 106f–107f
        full-thickness flap for uncovering of,
            111f–112f
        recession on, 171f
    mesial, 111f–112f
    midalveolar, 103–104, 104f
    supernumerary teeth as cause of, 104f
    temporary anchorage devices for movement
        of, 108
    tissue grafting for, 111
    uncovering of
        apically positioned flap for, 106, 108
        closed eruption technique for, 103–104
        full-thickness flap for, 111f–112f
    vertical, 104–106, 106f–107f
Mandibular molar impaction
    first molars, 141–145, 142f–144f
    second molars, 145, 146f–150f
Mandibular second premolar impaction
    autotransplantation for, 133, 134f–137f
    ectopic, 120f–121f
    illustration of, 115, 116f–119f
    lingual, 120f–121f
    palpation of, 115
    root development, 133
    uncovering of, 136f
Maxillary canines. *See* Labially impacted
    maxillary canines; Palatally impacted
    maxillary canines.
Maxillary central incisor impaction
    adverse sequelae of, 168f
    brackets for, 5
    ectopic labial, 6
    etiology of, 1–4, 2f, 4f
    gingival recession after improper surgery
        for, 168f
    high, 16
    horizontal
        apically positioned flap for, 7f–8f,
            166f–167f
        closed eruption technique for, 18f–19f
        relapse of, 166f–167f
        surgical replantation of, 20f–22f

a

labial
    apically positioned flap for uncovering of, 9f–10f
    closed eruption technique for, 15f–16f
    postoperative orthodontics for, 23
    preoperative orthodontics for, 5
    radiographic imaging of, 17f
    supernumerary teeth as cause of, 1–4, 2f, 4f, 12f
    uncovering of
        apically positioned flap, 6, 7f–10f, 23–24
        closed eruption technique, 11–19, 12f–19f
        excisional, 5, 6f, 23
        gingivectomy, 5, 6f, 23
        problems during, 23–24
        surgical replantation for, 20f–22f, 20–22
Maxillary lateral incisor crossbite, 31f
Maxillary molar impaction, 151, 152f
Maxillary premolar impaction, 131f–132f
Mesiodentes, 1, 3
Midalveolar impactions
    labially impacted maxillary canines
        apically positioned flap for, 51
        orthodontics for, 51
        uncovering of, 50
    mandibular canines, 103–104, 104f
    mandibular first molars, 143
Midcrestal incision, 11, 17
Molar impactions
    first, 141–145, 142f–144f
    mandibular. *See* Mandibular molar impaction.
    maxillary, 151, 152f
    second, 145–150, 146f–150f
Mucogingival junction, 34f, 38

**N**
Nasopalatine foramen, palatally impacted maxillary canines near, 73f–74f

**O**
Odontoma, 4
Orthodontic mechanics
    importance of, 163
    for labially impacted maxillary canines
        anchorage considerations, 53
        challenges, 55, 55f–59f, 58–59
        ectopic impaction, 51–53, 52f–54f
        midalveolar impaction, 51
    for premolar impaction eruption, 126, 129

**P**
Palatally impacted maxillary canines
    above apices of incisors, 88f–89f
    in adults, 88, 90f–91f, 92
    ankylosis of, 87, 92
    autonomous eruption of, 75, 92–93, 94f–95f
    bone loss caused by improper orthodontic mechanics in, 156f, 158f
    cervical headgear and, 72

closed eruption surgical technique for, 72–74
complex
    ankylosis of, 87, 92
    definition of, 75
    elastomeric chain for uncovering of, 81f–82f
    full-thickness flap for uncovering of, 87, 88f–89f
interceptive treatment of, 71–72
ligation of, tooth loss secondary to, 159f–160f
near nasopalatine foramen, 73f–74f
preorthodontic uncovering of
    in adults, 88, 90f–91f, 92
    advantages of, 92–93
    criticisms of, 93
    elastomeric chain for, 81f–82f
    esthetic results with, 93
    flap reflection for, 76–77, 77f–80f
    full-thickness flaps for, 77, 79f–80f, 83f–89f
    soft tissue punch for, 75, 75f–76f
    technique for, 75–92
    timing of, 94
prevalence of, 71
referrals for, 72
root resorption caused by, 96, 96f–99f, 161f
simple
    autonomous eruption of, 76
    definition of, 75
    examples of, 75f–80f
    flap reflection for uncovering of, 76–77, 77f–80f
    full-thickness flap for uncovering of, 77, 79f–80f, 83f–87f
    preorthodontic uncovering of, 75f–80f, 76–78
    soft tissue punch for uncovering of, 75, 75f–76f
spontaneous eruption of, 92
Pedicle flaps
    full-thickness
        illustration of, 61f
        mandibular canines uncovered with, 111f–112f
        palatally impacted maxillary canines uncovered with, 77, 79f–80f, 83f–87f, 87–88
        premolar impaction uncovered with, 119
    labially impacted maxillary canines uncovered with, 32f
    maxillary central incisor impaction uncovered with, 11, 32f
    split-thickness, 48, 49f
Pin, for uncovering labially impacted maxillary canine, 36f–37f
Premolar impaction
    autonomous eruption of, 130
    autotransplantation for, 133, 134f–137f
    in Down syndrome patient, 127f–128f
    eruption of
        ankylosis effects on, 130, 131f–132f
        autonomous, 130
        orthodontic mechanics for, 126, 129

extraction for, 138
horizontal, 116f
lingual, 129
mandibular second premolar
  autotransplantation of, 133, 134f–137f
  ectopic, 120f–121f
  illustration of, 115, 116f–119f
  lingual, 120f–121f
  palpation of, 115
  root development, 133
  uncovering of, 136f
maxillary, 131f–132f
midalveolar position, 115, 129
palatal position, 115
radiographic localization of, 115, 117f
root development, 133
root resorption caused by, 123f–125f
uncovering of
  closed eruption technique for, 119–125,
    120f–125f
  full-thickness flap for, 119
  gold chain for, 119, 122f
  preorthodontic technique for, 126,
    127f–128f

**R**
Recession
  on labially impacted and ectopically located
    mandibular left canine, 171f
  on labially impacted maxillary canines,
    164f–165f
Root resorption
  closed eruption technique and, 74
  labially impacted maxillary canines as cause
    of, 39f–41f, 58f–59f, 60, 64
  palatally impacted maxillary canines as cause
    of, 96, 96f–99f, 161f
  premolar impaction as cause of, 123f–125f

**S**
Second molar impaction
  mandibular, 145, 146f–150f
  maxillary, 151f–152f
Second premolar impaction. *See* Mandibular
  second premolar impaction.
Sequelae. *See* Adverse sequelae.
Simple palatally impacted maxillary canines
  autonomous eruption of, 76
  definition of, 75
  examples of, 75f–80f
  flap reflection for uncovering of, 76–77,
    77f–80f
  full-thickness flap for uncovering of, 77,
    79f–80f, 83f–87f
  preorthodontic uncovering of, 75f–80f,
    76–78

soft tissue punch for uncovering of, 75,
  75f–76f
Soft tissue punch, for uncovering palatally
  impacted maxillary canines, 75, 75f–76f
Split-thickness pedicle flap, 48, 49f
Supernumerary teeth
  extraction of, 3, 4f
  interceptive removal of, 3, 4f
  mandibular canine impaction caused by,
    104f
  maxillary central incisor impaction caused
    by, 1–4, 2f, 4f, 12f
Surgery
  appropriateness of, 163
  labially impacted maxillary canines treated
    with
    buccal object rule, 44, 46f
    cone beam computed tomography
      before, 44, 60, 61f
    location determinations before, 44
  replantation, maxillary central incisor
    impaction uncovered with, 20–22,
    20f–22f

**T**
Temporary anchorage devices, 108
Tissue grafting, 111
Tooth attachment, in closed eruption
  technique, 60
Tooth loss, 155, 159f–161f

**U**
Uncovering
  labially impacted maxillary canines. *See*
    Labially impacted maxillary canines,
    uncovering of.
  mandibular canine impaction. *See*
    Mandibular canine impaction,
    uncovering of.
  maxillary central incisor impaction. *See*
    Maxillary central incisor impaction,
    uncovering of.
  palatally impacted maxillary canines. *See*
    Palatally impacted maxillary canines,
    preorthodontic uncovering of.
  premolar impaction. *See* Premolar
    impaction, uncovering of.
  timing of, 163

**V**
Vertically impacted mandibular canines, 104–
  106, 106f–107f